D1622946

Type 2
Diabetes
Your Questions Answered

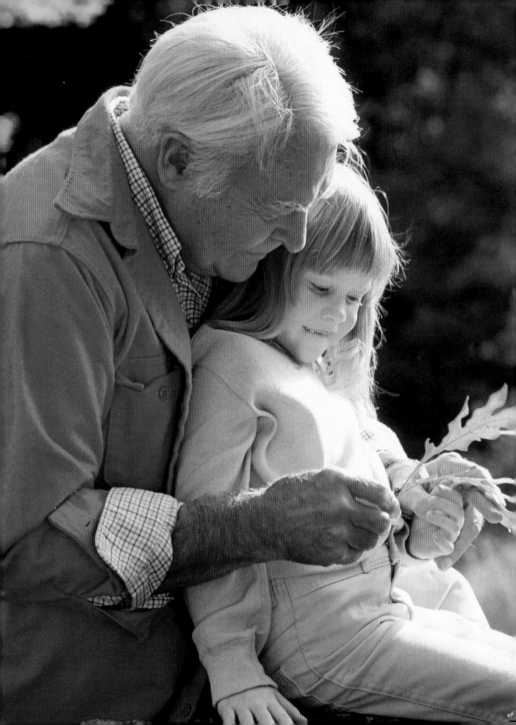

Type 2
Diabetes
Your Questions Answered

Rosemary Walker & Jill Rodgers

LONDON, NEW YORK, MUNICH, MELBOURNE, DELHI

Senior Editor Janet Mohun
Editors Kesta Desmond, Teresa Pritlove
Senior Designer Nicola Rodway
Designer Iona Hoyle
Managing Editor Adèle Hayward
Managing Art Editors Emma Forge, Karla Jennings
DTP Designer Julian Dams
Production Controller Heather Hughes

This edition first published in the United Kingdom in 2006 by
Dorling Kindersley Limited, 80 Strand, London WC2R 0RL
A Penguin Company

6 8 10 9 7 5
012-DD240-April/2006

Every effort has been made to ensure that the information in this book is accurate.
The information in this book may not be applicable in each individual case so you are therefore advised
to obtain expert medical advice for specific information on personal health matters. Never disregard
expert medical advice or delay in receiving advice or treatment due to information obtained from this
book. The naming of any product, treatment, or organization in this book does not imply endorsement
by the authors, imprimatur, or publisher, nor does the omission of such names indicate disapproval. The
publisher, authors, and imprimatur cannot accept legal responsibility for any personal injury or other
damage or loss arising from any use or misuse of the information and advice in this book.

Copyright © 2006 Dorling Kindersley Limited, London
Text copyright © 2006 Rosemary Walker and Jill Rodgers
The authors have asserted their moral right to be identified as the authors of this work.

All rights reserved. No part of this publication may be reproduced, stored in a retrieval system,
or transmitted in any form or by any means, electronic, mechanical, photocopying, recording,
or otherwise, without the prior written permission of the copyright owners.
All enquiries regarding any extracts or reuse of any material in this book
should be addressed to the publishers, Dorling Kindersley Limited.

A CIP catalogue record for this book is available from the British Library.

ISBN-13: 978-1-40531-150-2

Reproduced by Colourscan, Singapore
Printed and bound in China by Hung Hing

See our complete catalogue at
www.dk.com

**Based on text from Diabetes, A Practical Guide to Managing Your Health
by Rosemary Walker and Jill Rodgers, first published in 2004**

Foreword

We believe that understanding your diabetes and how it is treated is one of the most important factors in living successfully and healthily with the condition. In this book you will find up-to-date information about all aspects of living with Type 2 diabetes. We have answered many of the questions people commonly ask when they find out they have diabetes, from what they should be eating to how they should take their medication. In our answers we have offered clear, straightforward advice and information that is of practical use in everyday life.

Type 2 diabetes is a serious condition and it can affect you at any age and in any circumstances. Even if you don't have diabetes youreself, you may be affected by it because you live with someone or care for someone who has the condition.

We feel privileged to have written this book, and we hope you enjoy reading it and find the information interesting and useful. We wish you well on the journey of your life with Type 2 diabetes.

Jill Rodgers   Rosemary Walker

Contents

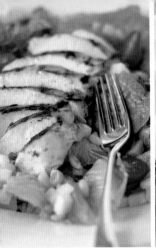
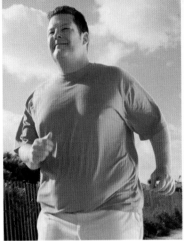
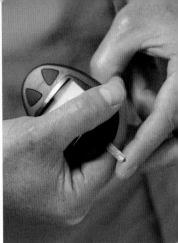

Living with diabetes

Medication

Long-term complications

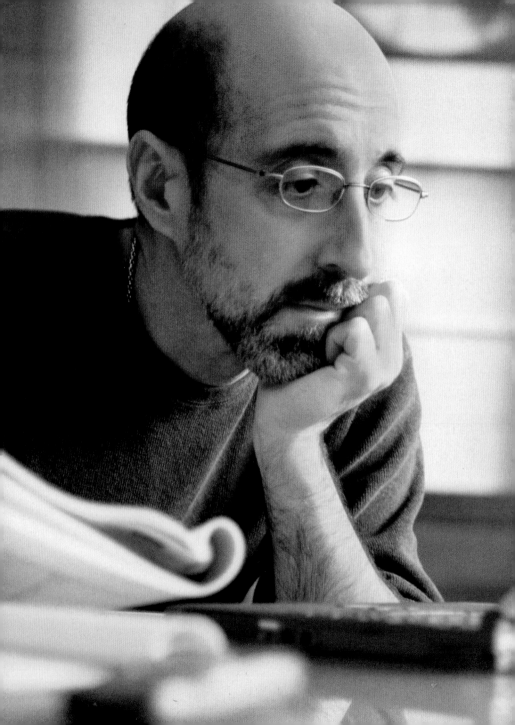

What is Type 2 diabetes?

Type 2 diabetes means your body cannot regulate your blood glucose, blood pressure, and blood fat levels properly. This can affect your short-term and long-term health, although a combination of treatment and lifestyle changes can help reduce these risks. In the past, Type 2 diabetes affected mainly older people but it now affects an increasing number of younger people.

Understanding diabetes

Q What is Type 2 diabetes?

Type 2 diabetes is the most common type of diabetes and used to be called "maturity onset" or "non-insulin-dependent" diabetes. When you have diabetes your body cannot use glucose (your body's main source of energy) in the usual way. Normally, glucose is absorbed by your body cells and burned as fuel. In Type 2 diabetes, glucose stays in your bloodstream because your natural supply of insulin – a hormone that regulates the level of glucose in your blood – is either not working properly or your body is not making enough of it. A raised blood glucose level can give you a range of symptoms including intense thirst and passing frequent or large amounts of urine. You are also much more prone to heart and circulatory problems because it is one part of a syndrome or collection of conditions that gives you high blood pressure and high blood fat levels. A high blood glucose level, without treatment, can damage your kidneys, nerves, and eyes. However, you can do a great deal to reduce the risk of these complications.

Q What is the difference between Type 1 and Type 2 diabetes?

People with Type 1 diabetes usually develop severe symptoms over a short time in childhood or early adulthood and their bodies cannot absorb any glucose without the help of a continuous supply of insulin either by injection every day (or an infusion of insulin through a pump). People who are prone to Type 1 diabetes have a specific genetic make-up that causes their bodies to destroy some of their own cells.

Is Type 2 less serious than Type 1 diabetes?

Definitely not. In some ways, Type 2 diabetes is a more serious condition than Type 1 because you could have it for a number of years before you are diagnosed. This means that you could already have developed some of the long-term complications of diabetes without being aware of them. In particular, Type 2 diabetes is linked with heart disease because of its association with high blood pressure and high cholesterol levels. These cause progressive thickening of your arteries over years that reduces your blood flow and increases the likelihood of your having a heart attack or stroke. Being overweight, particularly if you carry surplus weight around your waist, makes the risk of heart disease even greater.

Why does Type 2 diabetes develop?

There is no single reason why you develop Type 2 diabetes. A combination of factors affects how likely you are to develop the condition. Being overweight and inactive are two major factors that increase your risk of developing Type 2 diabetes. Other factors that put you at a higher risk of Type 2 diabetes include having a family history of diabetes and being a member of certain ethnic groups, such as South Asian, African, or Caribbean. See pp21–23 for more about the causes of diabetes.

How common is Type 2 diabetes?

Around 130 million people worldwide have Type 2 diabetes, and this number is increasing each year. In the UK, a total of 1.8 million people are known to have diabetes. Around 85 per cent of these have Type 2 diabetes. There are also many people who have Type 2 diabetes but have not yet been diagnosed with the condition.

Q Why is Type 2 diabetes becoming more common?

Today, people are much less active in their daily lives than those of previous generations, and this means they are more likely to be overweight or obese which, in turn, increases the risk of them developing Type 2 diabetes. More children and teenagers are also developing Type 2 diabetes for this reason.

Q What does insulin do in my body?

Insulin is a hormone (body chemical) that is made and released by your pancreas, which lies behind your stomach. Insulin acts like a key to let glucose (which comes from carbohydrate foods) move from your bloodstream into your cells where it is used to produce energy. Your body normally produces more insulin immediately and for some time after a meal, when there is more glucose around, and less at other times. Another hormone called glucagon (also produced by your pancreas) prevents insulin from letting your blood glucose level drop too low.

Q What would my blood glucose level be if I didn't have diabetes?

If you didn't have diabetes, your insulin and glucagon would keep your blood glucose level within a very narrow range (around 4–6 millimoles of glucose per litre of blood). As a result, whether you eat a lot of carbohydrate or only a little, your body has the constant supply of energy it needs in order to work properly.

Q How high can blood glucose rise in someone with Type 2 diabetes?

Very rarely, a blood glucose level of up to 100 millimoles per litre can be recorded when you are first diagnosed with diabetes. The most common situation is for your blood glucose to reach a level of 10–20 millimoles per litre – at which stage your symptoms would lead to you being diagnosed (see pp36–37).

What goes wrong in Type 2 diabetes?

Because your body doesn't produce enough insulin, produces it more slowly and/or your cells are resistant to the action of insulin (see below), your blood glucose cannot be as finely regulated as it would be normally. As a result, it is difficult for glucose to pass into your cells to be burned for energy, and so it builds up in your blood (see pp16–17).

What does insulin resistance mean?

This term means that, even if you still produce insulin, your body cannot use it in the normal way to let glucose into your cells. Insulin resistance is linked to you being overweight and being physically inactive. If you have Type 2 diabetes, you are also more likely to have high blood pressure and raised cholesterol levels.

How can I tell if I have Type 2 diabetes?

You may not have any symptoms, in which case your diabetes might only be found at a routine medical or eye test. Many of the symptoms you might experience can be part of growing older – for example, feeling tired, or getting up at night to pass urine – and you may not think you have diabetes, particularly if these symptoms are mild. You can read more about the symptoms of diabetes on pp34–35.

Will I have to inject myself with insulin every day?

Controlling your weight, eating healthily, and keeping or becoming physically active may keep your blood glucose level in the recommended range without any medication, sometimes for a short time or sometimes for years. If your blood glucose is regularly too high, even with your best efforts, you will be prescribed tablets and, eventually, you are likely to need insulin injections (see pp156–177).

Myth "Type 2 diabetes isn't serious unless you need insulin injections"

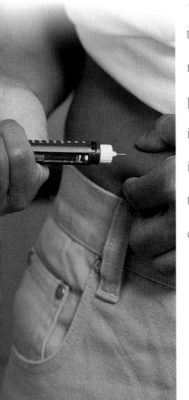

Truth The seriousness of diabetes isn't linked to the type of treatment you have but to whether measures such as your blood glucose and blood pressure are within healthy limits. For example, it's far more serious if your blood glucose level is too high and your tablets aren't controlling it than if your blood glucose level is under better control from taking insulin.

Why have I been told to control my weight?

Your weight influences how easy it is for your own insulin supplies to work properly and for your body to regulate your blood pressure. It also influences the type and dose of any medication you take. Being overweight can cause a rise in your blood glucose, blood pressure, and cholesterol levels, and it increases your risk of complications such as heart disease occurring. Keeping your weight within the recommended range for your height or, if you need to, losing some weight, has a number of health benefits.

Does Type 2 diabetes get worse over time?

Type 2 diabetes is a progressive condition. When this type of diabetes starts to develop, your body needs to produce more insulin to keep your blood glucose level in a healthy range. At first, healthier eating, losing weight, and increasing your physical activity may be sufficient to control your blood glucose level. Over time, however, your body probably won't be able to keep up with the demand for insulin – especially if you are overweight. Eventually, you are likely to need tablets and probably insulin injections to keep your blood glucose level between 4–7 millimoles per litre. Keeping your blood pressure in the recommended range is also important when you have Type 2 diabetes. You may need several types of tablet over time for this, too.

Can diabetes be cured?

As yet there is no cure for diabetes. The important thing is to actively manage your condition each day so that you can continue to live a healthy life. Keeping your blood pressure and blood cholesterol levels, as well as your blood glucose, in the recommended range can help prevent the long-term complications of diabetes.

How your body uses glucose

Glucose, in carbohydrate foods, is your body's main energy source. Without diabetes, the quantity of glucose in your blood is carefully regulated by two hormones produced by your pancreas. In Type 2 diabetes, this regulating system is impaired and the level of glucose in your blood rises too high. Over time, a high blood glucose level damages your eyes, kidneys, or nerves.

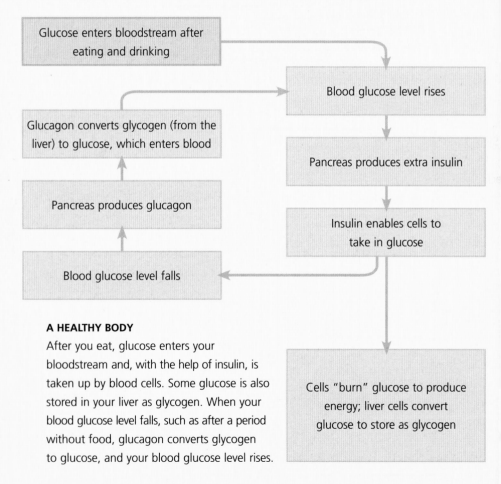

Glucose enters bloodstream after eating and drinking

Blood glucose level rises

Glucagon converts glycogen (from the liver) to glucose, which enters blood

Pancreas produces extra insulin

Pancreas produces glucagon

Insulin enables cells to take in glucose

Blood glucose level falls

Cells "burn" glucose to produce energy; liver cells convert glucose to store as glycogen

A HEALTHY BODY

After you eat, glucose enters your bloodstream and, with the help of insulin, is taken up by blood cells. Some glucose is also stored in your liver as glycogen. When your blood glucose level falls, such as after a period without food, glucagon converts glycogen to glucose, and your blood glucose level rises.

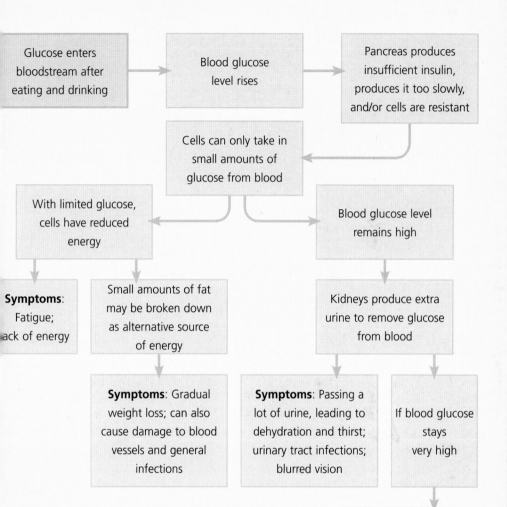

Glucose enters bloodstream after eating and drinking

Blood glucose level rises

Pancreas produces insufficient insulin, produces it too slowly, and/or cells are resistant

Cells can only take in small amounts of glucose from blood

With limited glucose, cells have reduced energy

Blood glucose level remains high

Symptoms: Fatigue; lack of energy

Small amounts of fat may be broken down as alternative source of energy

Kidneys produce extra urine to remove glucose from blood

Symptoms: Gradual weight loss; can also cause damage to blood vessels and general infections

Symptoms: Passing a lot of urine, leading to dehydration and thirst; urinary tract infections; blurred vision

If blood glucose stays very high

Symptoms: Extreme dehydration may develop leading to loss of consciousness

TYPE 2 DIABETES
Your pancreas produces insufficient insulin, produces it too slowly, or your body cells are resistant to it. Your blood glucose rises, and cells cannot burn glucose for energy. This leads to diabetes symptoms and, if your glucose level remains high, eventual damage to your eyes, kidneys, or nerves.

Type 2 diabetes and heart disease

Q What is the link between Type 2 diabetes and heart disease?

Type 2 diabetes is more than simply a raised blood glucose level. You are also likely to develop various problems related to your heart and blood vessels – for example, high blood pressure and high cholesterol levels. Although the link between high blood pressure and diabetes is not yet fully understood, it is thought that it may result from high levels of insulin circulating in your blood as a result of insulin resistance (which is usual in Type 2 diabetes). As a result, your blood vessels become scarred and hard plaques form – this causes narrowing of your blood vessels making it more difficult for your blood to flow. The risk of blockages in your blood vessels also increases; these can cause angina (severe chest pain) or a heart attack.

Q What is cardiovascular disease?

"Cardio" means heart and "vascular" means blood vessels. If you have Type 2 diabetes, you are prone to a range of cardiovascular problems including high blood pressure, hyperlipidaemia (a high level of fat in your blood), angina (severe chest pain), heart attack, stroke, peripheral vascular disease (pains in your legs when walking or resting due to reduced circulation), and heart failure. You are also two to five times more likely to develop cardiovascular disease (CVD) than someone without diabetes. CVD is one of the major problems associated with Type 2 diabetes.

How would I know if I have CVD?

CVD does not necessarily cause any symptoms and may only become apparent when you have a heart attack or a stroke. But it is possible for your health professional to look for signs of CVD, such as high blood pressure and high levels of cholesterol in your blood. If tests are positive, you can have treatment for these conditions even though they do not make you feel ill. This is why you need to have your blood pressure and blood cholesterol levels checked regularly.

Can I take drugs to prevent CVD?

Taking regular low doses of aspirin (or other blood-thinning tablets if you can't take aspirin) can help to reduce your risk. You may also be prescribed tablets to reduce your cholesterol level if you need them. Even if you need tablets, eating healthily and becoming or staying active will play an important role in lowering your risk of CVD.

What exactly are "raised blood lipids"?

When you have Type 2 diabetes, your levels of cholesterol and triglycerides – two types of lipids (fats) in the blood – are likely to be raised, a condition known as hyperlipidaemia. Both of these fats are essential in small amounts, but when their levels are raised they can damage your arteries (blood vessels). There are two types of cholesterol in your blood: high-density lipoprotein (HDL) and low-density lipoprotein (LDL). In a healthy person, there is a higher proportion of HDL to LDL, but when you have Type 2 diabetes, the reverse is often true. Treatment of raised levels of lipids in the blood aims to lower your blood fats and correct the ratio of HDL to LDL. This in turn prevents your arteries from narrowing.

Q How can losing weight prevent CVD?

If you are overweight, losing even a few pounds is one of the most important things you can do if you have Type 2 diabetes. Losing weight and becoming more active will help to lower your blood cholesterol levels and blood pressure. Your body will also become more responsive to the insulin you produce, and your heart will be under less strain.

Q Will physical activity help me prevent CVD?

Yes, just 30 minutes of moderate activity five times a week will help you to control your blood pressure and reduce your cholesterol level, which in turn reduces your risk of CVD. Physical activity helps you to lose weight because you not only burn more calories while you are active, but you also speed up your metabolic rate so that your body uses up more calories even when you are less active. See pp78–97 for how to become more active, whatever your activity level is now.

Q How important is it to stop smoking now I have Type 2 diabetes?

Very important: if you smoke, you have a far higher risk of CVD, heart attack, and stroke. Having Type 2 diabetes further increases the risk. Going to smoking cessation clinics and using nicotine replacement therapy such as patches or chewing gum can help you give up.

Q My Type 2 diabetes was diagnosed after a heart attack. How can I prevent another?

Taking any medication you have been prescribed to reduce your blood pressure and cholesterol level, increase your blood flow, and control your blood glucose level will make a big difference. Relaxation therapy and attending your cardiac rehabilitation meetings will help to reduce your risk. Stopping smoking and being active – for example, walking every day – are also important.

Causes of Type 2 diabetes

Is it possible to discover why I got Type 2 diabetes?

Type 2 diabetes develops as a result of a combination of factors, and it's not possible to know exactly why you have developed the condition. Some risk factors, such as being from a particular ethnic background and having a family history of diabetes, are genetic, and therefore beyond your control. Some factors, such as being overweight or inactive, may be the result of your lifestyle. Whatever your circumstances, your diabetes will not go away, but there is a great deal you can do to live with it successfully once you are diagnosed.

Can eating too much sugar cause diabetes?

Not directly. Sugar itself doesn't cause diabetes but eating sugary foods can make you gain weight, and being overweight can increase your risk of developing Type 2 diabetes. This is why making sure that your weight is in the correct range for your height can help to prevent Type 2 diabetes.

Could my Type 2 diabetes have been triggered by a viral infection?

No, only Type 1 diabetes can be triggered by a virus in a person who already has a genetic predisposition to diabetes (see p10). Type 2 diabetes is a different condition from Type 1 diabetes. Your diabetes may have appeared at the same time as you had an illness or viral infection, simply because your body produces extra glucose when you are ill, but you are unable to produce the extra insulin you need to deal with this. This means you develop a high blood glucose level and symptoms quite rapidly, and this in turn leads to you being diagnosed with diabetes.

Q Why does being overweight increase the risk of developing Type 2 diabetes?

Being overweight can make your body cells resistant to the action of the insulin that your body makes. Obesity, which is defined as weighing 20 per cent more than your ideal body weight, further increases your risk of Type 2 diabetes. Where you carry extra weight is also important. If you have excess weight around your waist (rather than your hips or thighs) your risk of developing Type 2 diabetes is even higher. See pp66–69 for more information on body shape and size.

DRUGS THAT INCREASE YOUR RISK OF DIABETES

Certain drugs for long-term conditions can raise your blood glucose level or prevent your insulin from working properly. If you take any of the following drugs, you have a higher chance of developing Type 2 diabetes. Rather than stopping your prescribed medication talk to your health professional about how to limit your risk.

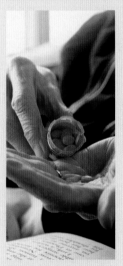

Steroids, such as prednisolone and dexamethasone. These are used to treat inflammatory conditions like chronic bowel conditions and rheumatoid arthritis. Taking steroids via an inhaler or skin patch will not affect your blood glucose in the same way that tablets and injections do.

Thiazide diuretics, such as bendroflumethiazide. These drugs remove excess fluid from your body. They may be prescribed to treat high blood pressure or heart failure.

Beta-blockers, such as propranalol, or vasodilators, such as diazoxide. These are often used for high blood pressure.

Immunosuppressants, such as cyclosporin. These are used to prevent rejection of organs following a transplant.

Q Why do some diseases make Type 2 diabetes more likely to develop?

Some diseases other than diabetes can affect how much insulin you make or can stop it working properly. Any of the following diseases put you at increased risk of developing Type 2 diabetes: pancreatitis (an inflammation of your pancreas); cystic fibrosis (a genetic condition that causes body secretions to be abnormally thick); and haemochromatosis (a build-up of excess iron that gradually damages your insulin-producing cells). There are also some hormonal disorders that can increase the risk of Type 2 diabetes developing. The main hormonal disorders linked with diabetes are Cushing's disease, in which your adrenal glands produce excess steroid hormones, and acromegaly, in which your pituitary gland overproduces growth hormone. These hormones prevent your insulin from working properly and this makes your blood glucose level rise.

Q Is there a link between pregnancy and getting Type 2 diabetes?

Yes. There is a type of diabetes known as gestational diabetes that can start during pregnancy. When you are pregnant, your body increases its blood glucose level to cope with the demands of your growing baby and, in turn, you need more insulin. If your body cannot produce enough insulin, your blood glucose level remains high and gestational diabetes is diagnosed. Once you have had gestational diabetes, you are at an increased risk of developing Type 2 diabetes because your body has shown that it has a tendency not to regulate your blood glucose levels. You can reduce the likelihood of getting Type 2 diabetes by taking regular physical activity and keeping your weight within the recommended range.

Who gets Type 2 diabetes?

Q Can you be born with Type 2 diabetes?

No, Type 2 diabetes is a condition that develops over time. It is most common in people over the age of 40, but there are increasing numbers of children and teenagers who are developing Type 2 diabetes, especially those who are overweight and inactive.

Q What are my chances of getting Type 2 diabetes if one or both of my parents has it?

If one of your parents has Type 2 diabetes, you are at a slightly increased risk of developing it; if both of your parents have it, your risk is much greater. If you have a strong family history of diabetes, you can do a lot to reduce your risk by keeping your weight in the normal range and becoming more active if you need to.

Q My sister has been diagnosed with Type 2 diabetes. Should I be tested for it?

If you have a brother or sister with Type 2 diabetes you have an increased risk of developing the condition. If you have an identical twin sister or brother who has Type 2 diabetes, you have a very high chance of developing it. Having a blood test will reveal whether you have Type 2 diabetes (see pp36–37). If you find you don't have diabetes, you can take steps to reduce your risk of developing it in the future.

Q I am overweight. Does this mean I will get diabetes?

Not necessarily, but being overweight can reduce your body's ability to regulate glucose levels, which in turn can lead to Type 2 diabetes. You can dramatically decrease your risk of Type 2 diabetes by losing weight. How your weight is distributed is also important. Carrying extra fat around your waist rather than your hips is linked with Type 2 diabetes (see pp66–69).

Is it true that ethnic background is a risk factor for Type 2 diabetes?

Yes, if you are of South Asian or African Caribbean descent, you have at least a five times greater chance of developing Type 2 diabetes than if you are of Caucasian origin.

I gave birth to large babies but didn't have gestational diabetes. Does this mean I won't get Type 2 diabetes?

One reason that babies grow very large is because they have to make more insulin to deal with extra glucose coming through the placenta. Even though you weren't diagnosed with gestational diabetes, finding out if any tests revealed an increased glucose level will help you and your health professional to assess your level of risk of Type 2 diabetes in the future.

RISK FACTORS FOR DEVELOPING TYPE 2 DIABETES

Your chances of developing Type 2 diabetes depend on a number of different factors, including your family background, your weight and body shape, and how much physical activity you take.

LOWER RISK	HIGHER RISK
Few or only one family member with diabetes	Many family members with diabetes
Caucasian	African Caribbean, or South Asian
No previous gestational diabetes (a form of diabetes that develops in pregnancy)	Gestational diabetes in the past
Fairly active	Very little activity every day
Normal weight for height	Overweight, especially around the waist

Type 2 diabetes and young people

Q Can children and teenagers develop Type 2 diabetes?

Yes, traditionally Type 2 diabetes has affected only older people but, with an increased tendency for children and teenagers to be overweight and less active, the incidence of Type 2 diabetes in this age group has increased dramatically in recent years, especially in North America and northern Europe.

Q How many young people are there with Type 2 diabetes?

It is estimated that there may be around 1,400 children in the UK with the condition. Children born today have a greatly increased risk of Type 2 diabetes and heart disease because of obesity and inactivity. It is likely that nearly half of all people diagnosed with Type 2 diabetes in the next 15 years will be young people.

Q Is Type 2 diabetes more or less serious if you develop it when you are young?

The condition is equally serious at whatever age it develops. However, the complications of diabetes are associated with the length of time you have it. So if you develop diabetes at a younger age, you are at greater risk of heart disease and the other complications of diabetes, such as eye, kidney, and nerve damage.

Q Do children grow out of Type 2 diabetes?

You cannot grow out of or be cured of diabetes. However, the risk of long-term problems associated with it can be greatly reduced by losing weight, if necessary, and being more active. These changes can make you better able to use the insulin that you produce naturally.

Q What's the best way to treat Type 2 diabetes in children and young people?

The ideal way is to help them to lose weight by encouraging healthy eating and being more physically active (see pp78–97). If these habits become a normal part of a child's lifestyle, they may delay the need for tablets and insulin injections, and make any prescribed medication as effective as possible.

Q My 20-year-old daughter has been diagnosed with Type 2 diabetes. What restrictions will she have on her life?

She will always need to look after her diabetes on a day-to-day basis, which she can do by eating healthily, staying active, and taking any medication she is prescribed. However, she won't be restricted in what she can do, unless she wants to pursue one of the few careers that have specific rules relating to people with diabetes (see p124).

Q What is MODY?

MODY stands for "maturity onset diabetes of the young", a rare type of diabetes that affects about 1 in 100 people with diabetes. It usually appears in your teens or 20s and is similar to Type 2 diabetes in that your treatment focuses on healthy eating and physical activity first, then tablet treatment and/or insulin if necessary. There are different forms of MODY, which might affect your risk of complications occurring, so having a genetic test (see below) is important.

Q I have had diabetes, which I treat with tablets, since I was 19. How do I know whether it is MODY or Type 2 diabetes?

MODY develops only in people with specific genes that cause a defect in the way the insulin-producing cells in your pancreas work. This leads to your producing less insulin. MODY can be confirmed by genetic testing. If several members of your family also developed diabetes at a young age, you can have the genetic test which will tell you what type of diabetes you have.

Long-term complications

Q **I've just been diagnosed with Type 2 diabetes. What sort of health problems might I develop in the long term?**

You are at increased risk of two main sets of complications: those affecting your heart and circulation (macrovascular problems) and those affecting your eyes, feet, kidneys, and nerves (microvascular problems). Although serious, these problems are not inevitable. You can do a lot to reduce the risk of them developing by leading a healthy lifestyle and working with your health professionals to ensure you have routine medical checks when you need them.

Q **How long after diagnosis do the complications of Type 2 diabetes usually occur?**

Complications take at least 5–10 years to develop but this can be misleading because you can have signs of them when you are first diagnosed. This is because you may have been developing Type 2 diabetes for years before your diagnosis. Once you know you have diabetes, you can slow the rate at which complications progress, or increase the time before they develop.

Q **What heart problems might I experience?**

Type 2 diabetes is strongly linked to high blood pressure and high blood cholesterol. These two factors increase your risk of cardiovascular disease (CVD) and heart attack (see pp180–183).

Q **Why is diabetes linked with kidney problems?**

High blood glucose levels over a period of years can damage the delicate filtering system in your kidneys (see pp188–189). If left untreated, this damage can eventually progress so that your kidneys no longer function efficiently. You will be offered urine tests once or twice a year to look for any early signs of damage.

Q Is it true that diabetes can affect my eyesight?

When you are first diagnosed with diabetes, you may have blurred vision. This is linked to high blood glucose levels and is usually temporary. Once your blood glucose levels reduce, your eyesight will return to normal. In the longer term, one of the complications of diabetes is retinopathy – damage to the small blood vessels at the back of your eye. Retinopathy can be successfully treated if diagnosed at an early stage, but if it is left untreated, your eyesight will be affected. Having your eyes checked at least once a year will tell you if you have retinopathy (see pp184–185).

Q Why are people with diabetes prone to foot problems?

Over a long period of time, high blood glucose levels can cause poor circulation and nerve damage, resulting in reduced sensation in your feet. This makes you more prone to problems such as ulcers on your feet or legs, or damage to the bones of your feet (see pp190–193).

Q How will having diabetes affect my sex life?

If you are a man, over time you may find it more difficult to get an erection because of damage to your nerves or circulation. There are a variety of treatments for erectile dysfunction (see pp196–197).

Q What can I do to prevent myself from getting the long-term complications of diabetes?

Controlling your blood glucose level and blood pressure as well as possible reduces your risk of complications. Eating healthily, being physically active, losing weight if you need to, stopping smoking, and taking prescribed tablets or insulin all help. Other important measures include attending your annual review and keeping your knowledge of diabetes up to date. To minimize foot problems, check your feet daily, and seek help if you notice any injuries or abnormalities (see pp190–193).

Reducing your risk of Type 2 diabetes

Q **Is it possible to prevent Type 2 diabetes?**

If you know that you are prone to diabetes because, for example, you have a family history of Type 2 diabetes or you had diabetes during pregnancy, making lifestyle changes can help you to delay or even prevent its onset. These changes include eating more healthily, becoming more active, and losing weight if you need to. Stopping smoking and drinking less alcohol do not affect whether or not you will develop diabetes, but they will help to reduce your risk of developing heart disease.

Q **How does keeping to the correct weight for my height help?**

It means that your body will be able to handle glucose and use insulin as efficiently as possible. If you are overweight, your resistance to insulin increases.

Q **Why is it important to stay physically active?**

Physical activity helps you to maintain your weight in the correct range for your height or to lose weight if you need to. It also increases your body's efficiency at storing and using glucose. Activity also keeps your heart and blood vessels healthy – this is very important if you are at risk of developing diabetes.

Q **Could I lose weight by changing my eating habits without taking more physical exercise?**

Yes, eating less is the key to losing weight. However, activity can go a long way to help. For example, you can burn off excess calories through activity. Reducing your calorie intake, and using more energy than you take in, will lead you to lose weight most successfully.

I am 50 and have been overweight for most of my adult life. Will losing weight now help me to prevent diabetes?

If you are overweight, losing weight will always improve your health, regardless of how old you are. There is no guarantee of preventing Type 2 diabetes, but being the correct weight for your height will greatly reduce your risk and will be of benefit if you do develop Type 2 diabetes.

I've always been slim. Will this naturally protect me from Type 2 diabetes?

Being the correct weight for your height is an important part of reducing your risk of Type 2 diabetes. However, body shape is also important; carrying extra fat around your waist rather than your hips increases the risk of diabetes. Checking your body mass index and waist size will help you to find out whether your weight and body shape are risk factors (see pp66–69).

There is a lot of diabetes in my family and we tend to be overweight. I want to protect my teenagers from diabetes but they eat a lot of junk food. What can I do?

Your children are at risk of Type 2 diabetes due to your family history, and their risk increases if they become overweight (too much junk food can cause weight gain, especially if your children are not very active). Share your concerns about Type 2 diabetes and the role high-calorie, high-fat, and junk food plays in weight gain. Including your children in the shopping for and preparation of food, adapting recipes (see p61), and helping them to learn about food labelling (see p53) may also help.

I am in my 60s and have Type 2 diabetes. How can I help my young grandchildren to avoid developing it?

Encouraging healthy eating habits by offering meals and snacks that are low in fat, salt, and sugar (reserving sweets and chocolate for special treats) will help to reduce their risk. You could also encourage them to walk rather than being driven short distances, or play active games rather than sit in front of a computer or television.

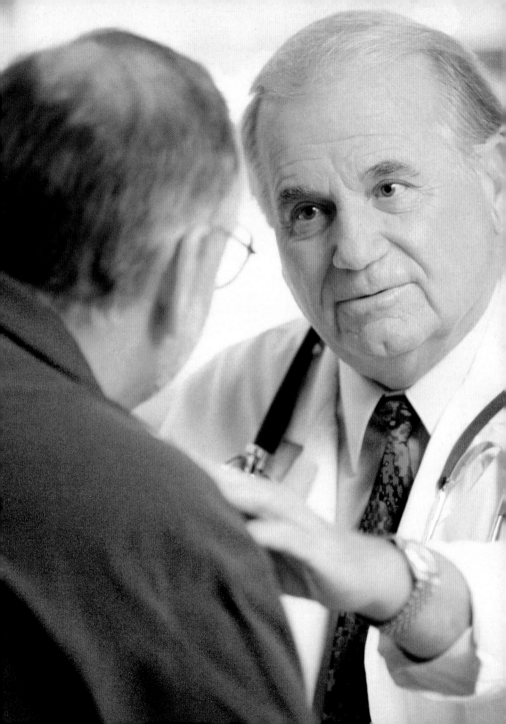

Finding out you have diabetes

You may be diagnosed with diabetes as a result of your symptoms; or you may have no symptoms and be diagnosed during a routine medical check. Discovering that you have diabetes can give rise to a range of emotions from anxiety and fear, to anger and guilt. A team of health professionals can give you help and support.

Symptoms of Type 2 diabetes

Q Could I have Type 2 diabetes even though I feel well?

Type 2 diabetes can sometimes be symptomless, and it may only be discovered when you have a routine medical or eye test which detects abnormalities. Equally, because Type 2 diabetes develops gradually, your symptoms may be mild and you may not notice them. If you think you may have Type 2 diabetes, ask your health professional about being tested.

Q I feel tired all the time, which I've been putting down to my age. Could I have diabetes?

Diabetes can cause tiredness if your body is unable to convert the glucose in your bloodstream into energy. Tiredness is a symptom of many conditions, but if you are also feeling thirsty and passing large amounts of urine, you may have diabetes – being tested will tell you whether this is the case.

Q Recently, I have been getting up several times a night to pass urine and feeling very thirsty. Does this mean I have diabetes?

Being thirsty and passing large amounts of urine are both symptoms of diabetes. When the level of glucose in your blood rises too high, your kidneys start to filter the excess glucose out of your blood and into your urine. As a result, you need to pass urine frequently, which you might notice particularly during the night. This makes you dehydrated, causing thirst and a dry mouth. If you drink sugary drinks to quench your thirst, this makes your blood glucose rise even higher. You then pass even more urine to get rid of the glucose and become even more dehydrated as a result.

I went to see my optician about blurred vision, and she suggested I have a test for diabetes. Why is this?

Blurred vision can be a symptom of diabetes. If your blood glucose level is high, the lenses of your eyes absorb glucose and water which makes them swell and affects your ability to focus properly. If you are diagnosed with diabetes and you reduce your blood glucose level, your lenses and your eyesight return to normal within a few weeks.

Is it true that cystitis and thrush can be a sign of diabetes?

Yes. When you have diabetes, the glucose in your urine provides an excellent environment for bacteria and fungi to grow and thrive, making cystitis (an inflammation of the bladder, usually due to bacterial infection) and thrush (a fungal infection of the vagina) more likely to occur frequently.

Do people with Type 2 diabetes get fruity-smelling breath?

Only people with Type 1 diabetes get this symptom because they have no insulin to process glucose, and their body has to break down fats instead to provide energy for cells. This process produces chemicals called ketones as toxic by-products. Ketones are partly excreted by the lungs, causing fruity-smelling breath.

If I have Type 2 diabetes without knowing about it, could I fall into a coma?

This is highly unlikely. However, a rare and serious condition called hyperosmolar non-ketotic syndrome (HONK) can sometimes lead to a coma. This develops gradually and makes you very dehydrated; you would have a very high blood glucose level and you would need to be treated in hospital. HONK usually happens if you are not well enough to detect the early symptoms of diabetes or if you have a very severe infection. If you suspect you have symptoms of diabetes, discuss this with your health professional.

Diagnosing Type 2 diabetes

Diagnosing Type 2 diabetes is straightforward and consists of tests to check the level of glucose in your blood. Initially, your health professional may use fingerprick blood tests and urine tests, both of which can detect the presence of glucose. However, neither test can diagnose diabetes conclusively as they cannot measure exact amounts of glucose, and you may need one or more further laboratory blood tests (see opposite). Sometimes one test is enough, but if results are inconclusive (for example, you may have symptoms of diabetes, but the test shows a normal blood glucose level, or you may have no symptoms and a blood glucose level that is slightly raised), you need further blood tests. A correct diagnosis ensures that you get the right treatment for your long-term health.

INITIAL MEDICAL TESTS

URINE TEST

A sample of your urine is tested using a dipstick that changes colour according to the amount of glucose present. The dipstick is then compared to a colour chart. The same test will also check for other substances present in your urine.

What the results mean If glucose is detected, or you have symptoms but no glucose, you will be referred for blood tests.

FINGERPRICK TEST

A drop of blood from your finger is placed onto a testing strip. This strip is then inserted in a blood glucose meter to be analysed.

What the results mean A healthy blood glucose level is in the range of 4–6 millimoles per litre. If your test result is above 6 millimoles per litre, or if you have symptoms, your health professional will suggest further blood tests (see opposite).

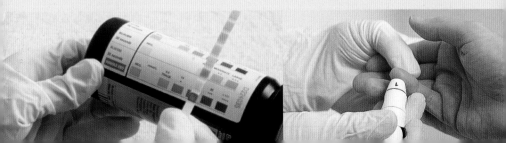

BLOOD TESTS TO DIAGNOSE DIABETES

Although urine and fingerprick tests can reveal a higher than normal blood glucose level, you need one or more of three laboratory blood tests to diagnose diabetes: the random or fasting blood glucose test and, if necessary, the oral glucose tolerance test.

RANDOM BLOOD GLUCOSE TEST

A blood sample is taken from your arm to send to a laboratory for analysis. The sample can be taken whether or not you have eaten. Your health professional receives the results within a week.

What the results mean If you have symptoms and a test result above 11.1 millimoles per litre, you are diagnosed with diabetes. If you have no symptoms, or the result is less than this, you may be asked to repeat the test while fasting or to take an oral glucose tolerance test.

FASTING BLOOD GLUCOSE TEST

You do not eat or drink overnight and a blood sample is taken in the morning. The sample is sent for analysis, and the results are available within a week.

What the results mean If you have symptoms and a test result above

7 millimoles per litre, you have diabetes. If you have no symptoms, or the result is less than this and you have symptoms, you may need to repeat the test or take an oral glucose tolerance test.

ORAL GLUCOSE TOLERANCE TEST

You do not eat or drink overnight. In the morning, a blood sample is taken before and 2 hours after drinking a sugary drink. The samples are sent for analysis and the results are available within a week.

What the results mean If your fasting level is above 7 millimoles per litre and/or your 2 hour test result is above 11.1 millimoles per litre, you are diagnosed with diabetes, whether or not you have symptoms. This test is used when other tests have been inconclusive or to diagnose gestational (pregnancy-related) diabetes.

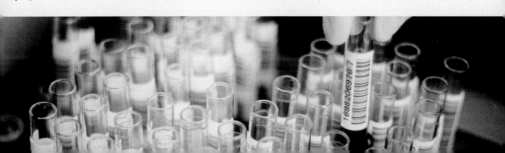

Dealing with emotions

Q **Is it true that my diabetes is caused by being overweight? I feel so guilty.**

It's true that being overweight makes your own insulin less likely to work properly. However, to develop Type 2 diabetes, you also need to be genetically predisposed to the condition, and you cannot control your genetic make-up. Many people feel responsible and guilty about what they have or have not done in the past. These feelings are normal, but focusing on looking after yourself now may help you feel more positive.

Q **I can't get used to the idea of having diabetes. Won't the tablets make it go away?**

Tablets for diabetes can lower your blood glucose level and make it seem as though your diabetes has disappeared, but it hasn't – you have diabetes for life. This can be a shock, and hard to accept, especially if your diabetes has come out of the blue and you haven't felt particularly unwell. Over time, feeling more in control will help you get accustomed to having diabetes. Talking to your health professional, family, friends, or other people, or contacting a support organization can help if you are having trouble adjusting.

Q **Can diabetes affect your mood? I feel very low about it and sometimes cry.**

Yes, having diabetes can affect your mood: it may be the worry of feeling unwell or thinking about your future health; the stress of having to think about food, activity, and blood glucose testing; or the frequent visits to health professionals or hospitals. If your mood is up and down, talking to your family and friends may help. If you still feel low or depressed most of the time, you may need treatment from your health professional. This could include counselling or antidepressant medication.

My partner says I've been really irritable since I got diabetes. Is it my blood glucose level?

A high blood glucose level can make you moody or irritable, but other causes include worry, feeling unwell, or even lack of sleep due to the need to go to the toilet during the night. Diabetes doesn't change your personality, but it can change the way you think and feel – working out what is making you irritable and explaining this to your partner or family can help.

I'm an optimist and I want to control my diabetes, not let it control me. How can I help myself?

Finding out as much as you can about which lifestyle changes will be beneficial to you and setting achievable short-term goals can help get you started. There may also be days when you feel less motivated. On these days, concentrating on the positive things that you can do to control your diabetes, such as healthy eating and physical activity, can help you cope.

I'm scared of going blind or needing an amputation. How can I deal with these fears?

These fears are understandable, especially if you know people who have these complications. Finding out how to prevent complications can help you to take positive action. Some concern about the future can be a good thing, but constant worry can have a negative impact on how you look after yourself. In this case, talking to someone about your worries can help reduce your fears.

Everyone seems to be nagging me about my food or my weight and it makes me cross. What can I do?

When you are newly diagnosed, it can be irritating to have other people suddenly commenting on what you eat and drink, especially if their opinions are ill-informed, judgmental, or out-of-date. People may do this because they care about what happens to you and want to help. Tactfully letting them know how their comments make you feel – and perhaps how they could help you more – might be useful.

Myth "Having diabetes gives you mood swings"

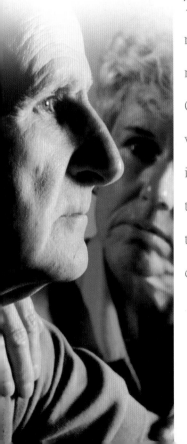

Truth Diabetes itself does not change your mood, but uncontrolled blood glucose levels can make you feel moody, irritable, or depressed. Other reasons for changes in your mood include worrying about your diabetes and how to control it, feeling unwell, or even lack of sleep due to the need to get up in the night to pass urine. At times, you may also have feelings of resentment, disappointment, or anger about your diabetes.

If I feel that I'm not coping, who could I talk to?

If you want to talk about a specific aspect of your diabetes, a diabetes helpline (see p202) can offer confidential and impartial information. If you feel you are not coping with your diabetes, your health professional can refer you to a counsellor. A local support group for people with diabetes – where you can share your feelings with others who understand what it is like living with diabetes – can also help.

How can I deal with the negative feelings I have towards my diabetes?

Strong negative emotions, such as fear, guilt, and anger are normal from time to time, especially when you are first diagnosed. Understanding as much as you can about diabetes and how to manage it can be helpful. Writing your feelings down (including any questions you have about diabetes care) can help make sense of them. Being regularly physically active can help to reduce stress. Discuss with your health professional any negative feelings you have.

I feel like diabetes has taken over my life. What can I do about this?

Adapting to life with diabetes can take a lot of thought, time, and energy. Eventually, blood glucose testing, healthy eating, being active, and taking tablets (or injecting insulin) will be more familiar. Understanding the importance of your diabetes-related tasks can help you to stay motivated. Sharing your experiences with others who have diabetes can also make it easier to cope.

My diabetes feels overwhelming and I can't face thinking about it. What can I do?

Breaking down your fears and anxieties into specific concerns, for example, about food or your blood glucose level, can help you. Tackle each concern one at a time. Learning as much as you can about Type 2 diabetes can help you feel in control.

Who's who in my healthcare team?

Q Who will help me to manage my diabetes?

You will be helped to manage your diabetes by a team of people trained in diabetes care, including a general practitioner (GP), practice nurse, dietitian, podiatrist, and an eye specialist who will take a retinal photograph (see p185). You may also see various other health professionals or care staff, such as district nurses, a diabetes specialist nurse, hospital consultant, and counsellor or psychologist. Ideally, one person will be your contact in between appointments.

Q I've been sent appointments for diabetes clinics at my GP surgery and the hospital. Which should I go to?

When you are first diagnosed, you may have some of your care at the surgery and some at hospital. For example, the hospital might run education sessions for people newly diagnosed with diabetes. Ask the staff in each clinic what the appointments are for and whether you need to go to both.

Q What's the difference between my practice nurse and a diabetes specialist nurse?

In general, practice nurses work in GP surgeries and health centres and are trained to run various clinics, including those for people with diabetes. Diabetes specialist nurses work only with people with diabetes and are often based in hospitals or diabetes centres, providing education for newly diagnosed people or those with specific difficulties. You may see your practice nurse most often and a diabetes specialist nurse occasionally, depending on your specific needs.

Q Will I see the same people at each appointment?

Not necessarily, although you will have one person who you can contact if you have difficulties about how your care is organized. It's likely that you will see a variety of health professionals who will support you in your day-to-day diabetes care and in the prevention of long-term complications.

Q What is an annual review?

At your annual review, your health professionals will assess how well your blood glucose level and blood pressure are controlled. They will also carry out a number of checks for the signs of the long-term complications of diabetes. It may be necessary for you to have some of these checks carried out more frequently than once a year. You can find out more about annual reviews on pp120–121.

Q Why would I need a psychologist to help with my diabetes?

When you have diabetes, you can have strong emotions which can get in the way of you looking after yourself. A psychologist can help you explore your feelings or can help with any specific issues that are causing difficulties with your diabetes care. If you are not sure why you have been asked to see a psychologist – or any other health professional – ask about it before or at the beginning of an appointment.

Q What happens to my appointments if I am in hospital?

If you know you have a diabetes clinic appointment at a time when you are going to be in hospital, you can let the clinic know in advance and change the time of the appointment. If you are in hospital unexpectedly, a relative or the hospital staff may need to cancel it on your behalf. You can make a new appointment when you are out of hospital.

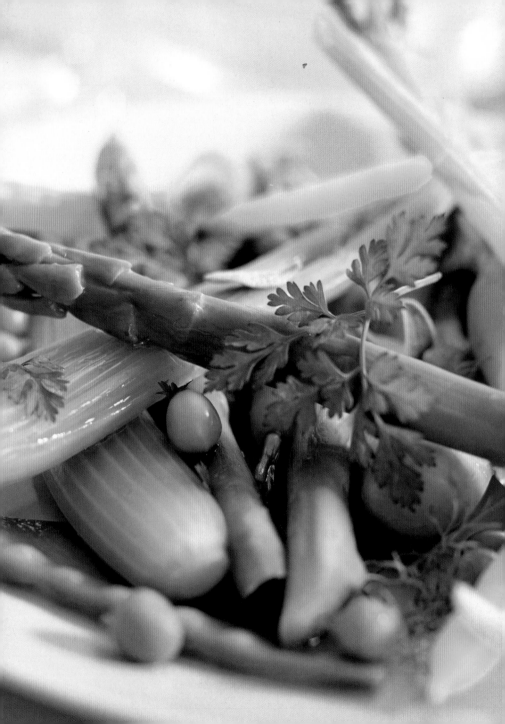

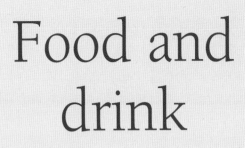

Food and drink

Eating healthily is one of the main ways in which you can manage your diabetes and help to keep your heart and blood vessels working efficiently. You may be overweight if you have Type 2 diabetes. If you want to lose weight, it's good to know which foods to choose to bring you success.

Types of food

Q What different types of food are there?

There are a number of main food types that, in combination, provide a healthy and balanced food intake. The chart opposite shows each food type and how it affects your blood glucose.

Q Why is it important not to eat too much salt, sugar, and fat?

Eating too much salt increases your risk of high blood pressure or makes high blood pressure worse if you already have it. Too much sugar can lead you to put on weight and can make it more difficult for you to control your blood glucose level. Fat is high in calories and eating more than the recommended amount can also cause you to put on weight. Eating too much saturated fat also increases your risk of heart disease.

Q What are antioxidants?

Antioxidants are a group of healing substances found in foods. Vitamins A, C, and E, beta-carotene and selenium – as well as many substances found in plants (phytochemicals) – have an antioxidant action. Eating foods that are rich in antioxidants has many health benefits, including protecting you from heart disease.

Q Can I take tablet supplements such as fish oils, vitamins, and minerals?

You can, but a balanced and varied food intake will provide all the nutrients you need to stay healthy. The only reason you might be advised to take supplements is if your healthcare team have diagnosed a deficiency. If you believe that you are deficient in a particular nutrient, your health professional will be able to discuss with you what action to take.

FOOD TYPES AND HOW THEY AFFECT HEALTH

FOOD TYPES	EFFECT ON GLUCOSE	RECOMMENDED INTAKE
Starchy foods: e.g. rice, potatoes, pasta, plantain, pitta bread	Your body's main source of energy. Different types affect your blood glucose in different ways (see p56).	Around two-fifths of each meal.
Sugars: e.g. sugar, honey, fizzy drinks	Sugary drinks and sweets raise blood glucose sharply. Sugar as part of other food has no more effect than other carbohydrate.	Take in moderation or after other food to reduce effect on blood glucose.
Proteins: e.g. meat, fish, eggs, beans, and pulses	Little effect on your blood glucose. Beans and pulses affect your blood glucose level slowly.	Up to one-fifth of each meal.
Fats: e.g. butter margarine, oils, ghee	Little effect on your blood glucose. Unsaturated fat (e.g. olive oil) is less harmful to your heart than saturated (e.g. butter). Excess fat can lead to weight gain and heart disease.	Up to 75g a day for women, 95g a day for men. Choose monounsaturated fat.
Dairy: e.g. milk and yoghurt	Milk and yoghurt contain carbohydrate and affect blood glucose level slowly.	Aim for three servings a day. A serving is one-third of a pint of milk or one small yoghurt.
Fruit, vegetables, and salads	Many fruit and vegetables are good sources of fibre, as well as containing important vitamins and minerals. Some fibre slows down carbohydrate digestion, so prevents blood glucose from rising too quickly.	At least five portions of fruit and vegetables through the day. Around two-fifths of each meal.

Healthy eating

Q What should I eat now that I have diabetes?

Healthy eating is the key to managing your diabetes. The principles of healthy eating for you are the same as those for everyone else. No foods are banned – but eating more of some foods and less of others can help to keep you healthy and your blood glucose level within the recommended range. Sometimes, you may not have a choice about what food is available but, generally, you can adapt recipes and meals so that you can enjoy food while still eating healthily (see p61).

Q How do I know whether I'm eating a healthy balance of food?

Selecting a balance of foods from the main food groups is the first step. Aim for starchy carbohydrates (such as wholegrain bread and cereals, pasta, rice and potatoes) to make up about a third of what you eat, with fruit and vegetables forming another third. Making up the rest of your food intake from lean protein foods and low-fat dairy products will give you a healthy balance. Choosing lower fat alternatives where you can will help to reduce your risk of heart disease.

Q Does it really matter what I eat? My health professional has told me I'll eventually need to take tablets – and probably insulin – anyway.

Eating healthily is not simply about avoiding medication to treat your diabetes – it reduces your risk of heart and circulatory diseases, helps your digestive system to work more effectively, and helps your pancreas be more efficient if it is struggling to produce enough insulin. Type 2 diabetes is progressive and you may need tablets and insulin in time, but eating healthily can help slow down this progression and make it easier to manage your blood glucose level.

I'm vegetarian and have Type 2 diabetes. Does this make any difference to what I should eat?

Healthy eating principles for diabetes remain the same whether you are vegetarian or following any other eating pattern. Vegetarian eating is not necessarily lower in fat just because it doesn't include meat. Replacement proteins such as cheese can also be high in saturated fat. Knowing this will help you choose more healthy protein options. There is no difference in the amount or type of carbohydrate you need to eat.

My local supermarket seems to label every food as healthy – how can I tell if they are?

Many supermarkets now sell ranges of food that are healthier than their counterparts. It could mean the food is healthier in only one aspect or several – for example, less fat, less sugar, fewer calories, or more fibre, or it could include a range of more healthy aspects. Reading the label (see p53) will help you work out which foods might help you reach your healthy eating goals. In general, processed foods will still be less healthy than those you prepare using fresh ingredients.

Do I need to eat special diabetic foods?

No. Foods labelled "diabetic" are often expensive and do not give you any benefits. They usually contain a sweetener called sorbitol, which is high in calories and still makes your blood glucose level rise. In large quantities, sorbitol can give you diarrhoea.

Should I use intense (artificial) sweeteners?

You can use intense sweeteners as an alternative to sugar to sweeten food and drinks, such as tea and coffee. These products contain aspartame, saccharin, cyclamate, acesulfame K, or sucralose, none of which will affect your blood glucose. These products are classed as food additives and, for this reason, have been tested for safety.

Myth "People with diabetes can't eat sugar"

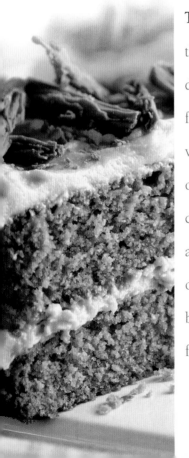

Truth It's the amount and type of sugar in food that are important to think about when you have diabetes, rather than sugar itself; even nutritious foods that are recommended, such as fruit, vegetables and milk, contain a certain amount of sugar. More obviously sugary foods such as cakes and sugary drinks aren't recommended on a regular basis for anyone, but even eating these occasionally won't have a lasting effect on your blood glucose level. If you have a hypo, sugary foods and drinks are the treatment you need.

Choosing healthier options

Which carbohydrate-containing foods are better for me?

Starchy carbohydrates with each meal, for example grainy bread, pitta bread, pasta, basmati rice, noodles, bulgar wheat, rice, oat and wholegrain and cereals are better for you as they take longer to digest and therefore help your blood glucose level stay more even.

I know that protein doesn't really affect my blood glucose, so does it matter what type I eat?

Protein foods low in fat, such as semi-skimmed milk, low-fat yoghurt and cheese, beans, peas, and lentils, will help reduce your risk of heart disease. Eating oily fish such as mackerel or salmon twice a week and choosing leaner cuts of meat will also protect your heart.

I'm trying to cut down on how much fat I eat – what can I do to make this easier?

You can reduce your fat intake by choosing foods such as low-fat spreads, crème fraîche and Greek yoghurt, or low-fat fromage frais instead of yoghurt or full-fat cream. White fish, which is lower in fat than meat, and leaner cuts of meat will also help. Grilling meat instead of frying, and draining excess fat during cooking are other ways of cutting down on fat. Avoiding processed foods and fried or pastry-based snacks will also help.

How can I make sure I eat at least five portions of fruit and vegetables every day?

Adding extra fruit to breakfast cereals and yoghurts, including a glass of fruit juice or a side salad with a meal, and having fruit and raw vegetable snacks instead of fatty foods will increase your fruit and vegetable intake. You can also add beans or vegetables to dishes such as shepherd's pie and chilli con carne. Frozen and tinned versions are easy to prepare and still count towards five a day.

Q I have high blood pressure and need to cut down on salt, how can I do this?

Most processed and convenience foods (including stock cubes and soy sauce) tend to be high in salt, so cutting down on these can help to reduce your salt intake. Reducing the amount of salt you add to your meals, either while you are cooking or at the table, will also reduce your overall salt intake.

Q How can I make sure that when I eat dried or fruit juice my blood glucose doesn't rise too high?

The carbohydrate (fructose) in fruit and fruit juice will make your blood glucose level rise. Limiting yourself to small amounts, including dried fruit and fruit juice with a meal and spacing out your fruit intake throughout the day will give you the nutritional benefits without raising your blood glucose too high.

Q Which drinks will make my blood glucose level go up?

Sugary drinks such as glucose drinks, cola, lemonade, and orange juice are digested very quickly and can cause a sharp rise in your blood glucose level (which is why it is recommended that you drink them when your blood glucose is too low). Sugar added to tea or coffee will have the same effect. Because your body is unable suddenly to increase its insulin production when you have Type 2 diabetes, your blood glucose may take some time to return to an acceptable level.

Q Which drinks won't affect my blood glucose level?

For day-to-day drinks, water or sugar-free drinks such as diet cola won't affect your blood glucose level. Tea, coffee, and other hot drinks without added sugar will not affect your diabetes. Drinking them with skimmed or semi-skimmed milk will ensure their fat content is not too high. Powdered drinks can have a high fat content, so checking the label will help to you identify the healthier low-calorie options.

Reading a food label

Labels on food items can give you useful information to help guide your food choices. When checking a food label you will find that ingredients are always listed in decreasing order of weight. Most labels give information based on values per 100g and per serving.

Energy Written as kilojoules (kj) and kilocalories (kcals), usually shortened to calories – this information can help if you are calorie counting to lose weight. Generally, opt for low-calorie products.

Protein Protein is unlikely to cause any large fluctuations in your blood glucose level.

Carbohydrate The total amount of carbohydrate is given, and sometimes also how much of it is made up of sugars (2g or less of sugar per 100g is low). This can help you to determine the affect of that food on your blood glucose level.

Fat Choosing items with a lower fat content (3g or less per 100g is low) will help you to lose weight. Foods with a higher proportion of mono- or polyunsaturated than saturated fats are healthier.

Fibre Choosing foods with a higher fibre content will help keep you healthy.

Sodium This is the salt content, and limiting your intake will be beneficial to your blood pressure.

NUTRITION INFORMATION

Typical values	per 100g	per half can
Energy	464kJ 109kcal	545kJ 129kcal
Protein	7.1g	8.3g
Carbohydrate of which sugars	18.9g 2.0g	22.2g 2.4g
Fat of which saturates	0.6g 0.1g	0.7g 0.1g
Fibre	5.2g	6.1g
Sodium	0.2g	0.2g

PER HALF CAN 129 calories, 0.7g fat of which 0.1g saturates

When to eat

Q Should I eat at strict times?

No, but if you know when your tablets or insulin work, you can ensure your meals or snacks coincide with these times – your health professional will help you to identify when this is. For example, some tablets may make your blood glucose level drop mid-morning or mid-afternoon, in which case you might need to eat a snack at these times to compensate. If you can't eat when you need to, perhaps because of long shifts or meetings at work, talking with your health professional will help you find out about different medications that may suit your routine better.

Q Why is it important for me to eat regular meals?

Regularly eating meals containing carbohydrate will give you energy, help your digestive system to function properly, and help avoid sharp rises and falls in your blood glucose level. Regular meals also prevent you needing additional snacks to compensate for meals you have missed, so they help to control your weight. A regular eating pattern is also more likely to fit in with any tablets or insulin that you take for your diabetes.

Q I normally eat one large meal a day – is that alright?

Having only one large meal a day is not the best way to balance your blood glucose levels or control your appetite. Your body may struggle to use all the energy this meal provides, which could contribute to increasing your weight. Your body will also be deprived of energy at other times of day when you are not eating. Your blood glucose level, and whether you have hypos, will tell you if your eating pattern is suiting your diabetes.

Should I have snacks during the day?

Not everyone needs to, but if you inject insulin or take insulin-stimulating tablets, you may find that you need a snack around the time when your insulin or tablet is having its peak effect (see p158 and p167). If this is the case for you, making sure that your snacks are low in fat will help to prevent you putting on weight.

If I get hungry between meals, what should I snack on?

Vegetables, plain popcorn, low-fat yoghurts and milkshakes, and fresh and dried fruit are healthy snacks. They are lower in calories and contain beneficial vitamins and minerals. Having a variety of these snacks throughout the day, if you need them, will help your blood glucose to stay balanced.

What is the maximum time I should leave between meals?

There is no maximum time, but you may find that you get hungry if you leave long gaps between meals, which might tempt you to eat unhealthy snacks or larger meals, which can then cause your blood glucose level to rise. Making your mealtimes fit both your daily routine and any blood glucose lowering medication you take is more important than the exact time between meals.

What happens if I am fasting?

When you go without food, you may need to adjust the dosage of your tablets or insulin for both the period that you are fasting and the times that you are eating. Talking with your health professional will help you work out what will best suit your circumstances.

It seems like I'll be eating more now I have diabetes. I'm already overweight – what can I do?

Rearranging the times and amounts you eat rather than eating more, can help you to lose or not put on weight. Choosing lower-fat foods in general, and low-calorie alternatives as snacks, will also help keep your weight under control. See pp70–75 for more help on losing weight.

Carbohydrates and the glycaemic index

Q Why are carbohydrates important in Type 2 diabetes?

Carbohydrates, also known as sugar, starch, and fibre, are broken down into glucose when they are digested, and insulin then helps that glucose move into your cells to be used for energy or stored for use later on. If you have Type 2 diabetes, your body is resistant to insulin so the glucose stays circulating in your blood. You need carbohydrate-rich foods for energy, but choosing carbohydrate foods that your body digests at a slower rate will help to reduce the demand on your insulin and so keep your blood glucose level more stable.

Q Which carbohydrates are digested quickly?

Carbohydrates like glucose, sugary drinks and white bread are digested easily and rapidly. They cause your blood glucose level to rise sharply, resulting in an immediate demand for insulin. You don't need to avoid them, but eating them with other foods – for example, eating bread as a sandwich, slows down their absorption so that they don't have a dramatic effect on your blood glucose.

Q Which carbohydrates are digested slowly?

Pasta, noodles, basmati rice, grainy bread, beans and pulses are broken down into glucose relatively slowly during digestion. They do not raise your blood glucose sharply, so eating them helps to keep your blood glucose level balanced.

I've heard that some people with diabetes count their carbohydrates. What is this and would it be useful for me?

Carbohydrate counting is one way of assessing how much carbohydrate you are eating. Many people with Type 1 diabetes use this method to calculate the dose of insulin they need. If you have Type 2 diabetes, it may help to know how much carbohydrate you are eating so that you can ensure your food intake remains balanced. If you have Type 2 diabetes that is treated with insulin, factors such as how resistant your body cells are to the action of insulin, mean that assessing carbohydrate on its own will not tell you how much insulin you need. If you want to learn more about assessing carbohydrate intake and whether it could help you, consulting your health professional may be a useful step.

UNDERSTANDING CARBOHYDRATE CONTENT

The more carbohydrate your food contains, the more insulin you need to convert it into immediate or stored energy. Knowing how much carbohydrate is in different foods can help you understand its effect on your blood glucose level.

AMOUNT	EXAMPLES OF TYPE OF CARBOHYDRATE
10g	1 thin slice bread, 1 tablespoon uncooked rice, 1 digestive biscuit, 2 tablespoons baked beans, 1 small apple
15g	1 medium slice bread, 1 90g boiled potato, 7–10 medium chips, 1 crumpet, 1 medium sausage roll, 1 medium grapefruit
20g	1 thick slice bread, 1 large croissant, 1 cup custard, 1 mango, 2 tablespoons raisins
30g	1 bagel, 1 large scone, 1 cup bran cereal, 1 jam tart, 4 slices pineapple, 8–10 dried apricots

Q How does the glycaemic index work?

The glycaemic index (GI) is a ranking of carbohydrate-containing foods based on the length of time they take to make your blood glucose level rise. Pure glucose has a rating of 100 and all other carbohydrate foods are rated in relation to this. Foods digested slowly have a low GI rating (below 55), medium foods are rated between 55 and 70, and foods that are quickly absorbed have a high rating of 70 or above.

Q Should I eat high or low GI foods?

Because low GI foods are more slowly absorbed, they produce a slower rise in your blood glucose level than those with a high GI rating. Trying to include at least one low GI food at each meal will balance the effect of foods that have a higher GI rating and means you don't need to avoid all high GI foods.

Q Why do similar foods have a different GI rating?

If a high GI food is combined with fat, the GI is lowered. This is why chips and sautéed potatoes have a lower GI than potatoes cooked without fat. The way that food is cooked also influences the GI rating. For example, a cooking method such as baking breaks down the starch molecules in potatoes to a greater degree than boiling. This factor raises the GI rating and explains why jacket potatoes have a higher GI than boiled potatoes.

Q How does eating a combination of foods affect GI ratings?

The GI rating of a particular food only tells you how quickly or slowly it raises blood glucose when eaten on its own. You usually eat a mixture of foods at any one meal – bread is often eaten with butter or margarine, and potatoes with meat and vegetables, for example. Combining foods with different GI ratings changes the overall GI of a meal.

Q How can I apply the glycaemic index to the food I eat in my everyday life?

You can use it as a guide to which low GI foods to include in a meal or snack. If you eat a baked potato (high GI), for example, adding baked beans (low GI) reduces the overall GI of the meal, and so the effect on your blood glucose is less. Low GI foods also tend to be more filling, making you less hungry between meals.

GLYCAEMIC INDEX OF COMMON FOODS

Foods have a GI rating between 1 and 100. Glucose (sugar) is 100 because it causes blood glucose to rise rapidly – within 30 minutes of eating. Different foods need to be specifically measured for their GI rating (individual brands of the same food can vary). These are some foods that tend to fall into the different categories of GI.

LOW (BELOW 55)
- Fruit: apples, grapefruit
- Vegetables: all pulses, such as chickpeas, kidney beans; sweet potatoes
- Cereals and grains: porridge with milk, rolled oats, oat bran, pumpernickel, basmati rice, wheat tortilla, pasta, instant noodles
- Snacks and desserts: peanuts, milk chocolate, yoghurt
- Beverages: milk

MEDIUM (55–69)
- Fruit: melons, pineapples
- Vegetables: sweetcorn, beetroot, new potatoes
- Cereals and grains: muesli, instant porridge, grape nuts, wholemeal bread, rye bread, croissants, brown rice, couscous
- Snacks and desserts: digestive biscuits, muesli bars, full-fat ice-cream
- Beverages: cranberry juice

HIGH (70 OR ABOVE)
- Fruit: dates, watermelons
- Vegetables: parsnips, broad beans, mashed potatoes, baked potatoes
- Cereals and grains: cornflakes, puffed rice cereal, wheat biscuit cereal, bagels, brown/white bread, instant rice
- Snacks and desserts: rice cakes, jelly beans, doughnuts
- Beverages: glucose drink

Healthier cooking

Q How can I cook food to make it low in fat?

Grilling, steaming, microwaving, or baking foods rather than frying them reduces their fat content. Placing meat on a rack in the oven helps to drain away excess fat.

Q If a recipe states frying as a cooking method, what should I do?

Consider whether you could use one of the above methods instead. Or, if you do fry food, using the smallest amount of monounsaturated oil, such as rapeseed oil, is the healthiest way.

Q I love eating sweet puddings. How can I still enjoy them without putting on weight?

Using a small amount of intense (artificial) sweeteners can sweeten a dish more effectively than a large amount of sugar. This will help reduce the calorie content, but puddings are often high in fat too so having smaller quantities or eating them less often will reduce the effect they have on your weight.

Q I've started eating more vegetables because they're low in calories. How can I stop my meals becoming too bland?

Adding ginger, garlic, or other spices to a vegetable dish or sprinkling herbs such as basil, tarragon, rosemary, dill, sage, mint, thyme, or oregano on vegetables all help to bring out their flavour and mean that you are less likely to add salt. Low-fat dressings and marinades on your food also give a variety of tastes.

Q I find it difficult to cut down on cheese, even though I know it's high in calories. What can I do?

Lower fat (and therefore lower calorie) varieties of most cheeses are available, but they are still high in fat. Eating smaller amounts of strong-tasting cheese gives you the same taste with fewer calories. Parmesan, for example, is high in fat, but has a very strong flavour – you need far less than you would of most other cheeses.

HOW YOU CAN ADJUST RECIPES

Soups	Using more vegetables will increase fibre content. Fat content can be reduced by adding low-fat yoghurt rather than cream.
Cheese-based starters	Try using goat's cheese or feta cheese, which have a lower fat content than cheese made from cow's milk.
Savoury nibbles	Lightly brush oil onto spring rolls, filo pastry snacks, or cheese in breadcrumbs, and bake rather than deep-fry them.
Mince dishes	Pre-cook beef or lamb mince to drain off some of the fat. Meat substitutes or soya both contain less fat.
Pies	Use a very thin layer of pastry or make a potato topping instead of pastry; try adding herbs or chopped spring onions to a mashed potato topping as an alternative to butter.
Casseroles	Replace a proportion of the meat in a recipe with vegetables.
Pasta dishes	Tomato-based sauces are healthier than cream-based sauces.
Mayonnaise	Try a combination of natural yoghurt and half-fat crème fraîche instead of mayonnaise, which is high in fat.
Tiramisu	Try making this with virtually fat-free fromage frais and reduced-fat cream cheese in equal quantities instead of eggs and mascarpone cheese. You can still add a small amount of sugar.
Cheesecake	Opt for low-fat soft cheese, add fresh fruit, and decorate with grated orange or lemon rind rather than cream.
Crumble	Use porridge oats for the crumble, and use more fruit filling and less crumble topping.
Custard	Use skimmed or semi-skimmed milk rather than full-fat milk, and instead of using sugar, add an intense (artificial) sweetener.

Eating out

If you are eating out, many restaurants now offer healthier options, which are lower in fat, sugar, and calories, and smaller portions. Also, keeping to one or two courses can help you to eat more healthily.

If no healthy options are available, or you feel like eating less healthily for once, and you inject insulin, you can adjust your dose to accommodate a rise in your blood glucose level if you need to. If you don't have this option, your blood glucose will rise temporarily, but will fall once you get back to your usual eating pattern.

If you often eat out, selecting your food with care can help you to eat healthily. When choosing a starter from the menu, a fruit- or vegetable-based dish is healthier than anything that is deep-fried or drenched in sauce or oil. For your main course, baked

MEAT DISHES

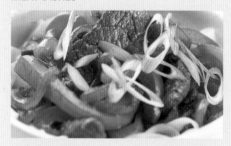

Good choices: Steak without sauce; roast chicken (with skin removed); grilled lamb steak (with fat removed); stir-fried pork with vegetables.

Less good choices: Beef stroganoff; steak and kidney pie; steak in creamy sauce; fried lamb chops; burger in a bun.

FISH DISHES

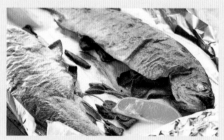

Good choices: Baked or poached salmon or tuna; grilled swordfish steak; smoked mackerel fillets; tuna salad; potato-topped fish pie.

Less good choices: Fish in batter; deep-fried scampi; fish in creamy sauce; fish in cheese-based sauce.

or boiled potatoes without butter are healthier than roast, sautéed, and mashed potatoes. Asking for extra vegetables and less meat, and requesting that any sauces are brought in a separate jug, means you can control how much goes onto your plate. To finish, fresh fruit or fruit-based desserts, or sharing a pudding with a friend can help you to eat fewer calories.

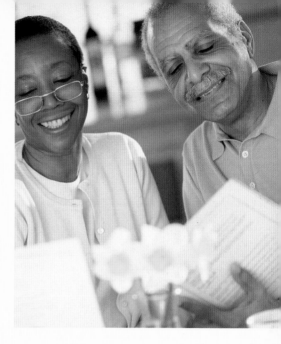

PASTA DISHES

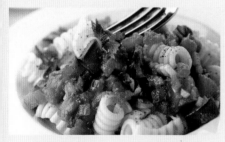

Good choices: Pasta with vegetable or tomato sauce; spaghetti bolognese; pasta with tuna or smoked mackerel; seafood pasta.

Less good choices: Pasta with creamy sauce, such as carbonara; beef lasagne, pasta with four-cheese sauce.

VEGETABLE-BASED DISHES

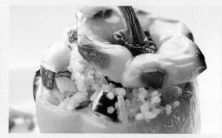

Good choices: Vegetable-stuffed peppers; vegetable stir-fry; spanish omelette; steamed vegetables with rice; ratatouille; grilled vegetable kebabs.

Less good choices: Vegetable pizza; cauliflower cheese; vegetable samosas; vegetable pasty.

Alcohol

Q Is it safe to drink alcohol?

There is no reason why you shouldn't drink alcohol when you have diabetes, unless you have been advised not to because of other medical conditions or treatment.

Q How much alcohol can I drink?

The standard guidelines for alcohol consumption are the same for you as for the general population: women can drink up to two units a day and men can drink up to three units daily (see box opposite).

Q Why might I get a hypo if I drink a lot?

When you drink alcohol, your blood glucose level rises initially because alcohol contains carbohydrate. As you continue to drink, your liver's ability to produce glucose is reduced and your blood glucose may start to fall. If you take insulin or insulin-stimulating tablets you may have a hypo (hypoglycaemia; see pp126–127). You can reduce this risk by having a meal or snacks containing carbohydrate before or while drinking and also afterwards.

Q Can I adjust my tablets or insulin injection if I know that I'm going out for a drink?

If you know you will be drinking alcohol and food may be in short supply, you may want to take a smaller dose of your tablets or insulin on that day to reduce the risk of a hypo. Carrying a snack with you as well as your usual hypo remedies might be helpful, too.

Q I'm trying to lose weight. Should I avoid alcohol?

Alcohol is high in calories, so cutting down can help you to lose weight or prevent weight gain. It also helps to drink low-calorie mixers with your alcoholic drinks: conventional mixers, such as tonics, colas, lemonade, and fruit juices are high in sugar.

I'm going to an office Christmas party and everyone will be drinking heavily. How can I stay in control?

Having a meal beforehand or eating snacks while and after you are drinking will lessen the effect of the alcohol. Substituting glasses of water for some alcoholic drinks can help and will mean that you still have a drink in your hand. It will also help if someone else knows what to do if you have a hypo. People who don't know you might think you are intoxicated when in fact you are hypo – and they won't necessarily realize that you need help quickly.

ALCOHOL AND BLOOD GLUCOSE

Alcoholic drinks contain carbohydrate and will initially raise your blood glucose level. However, in larger quantities, alcohol prevents your liver from releasing glucose, so it can lower your blood glucose and increase the risk of you having a hypo.

POINTS TO REMEMBER ABOUT ALCOHOL

Drinking a lot of alcohol can cause hypoglycaemia if you are taking insulin or insulin-stimulating tablets so be prepared and learn to recognize signs of a hypo (see pp126–129).

Drinking alcohol with a meal or some carbohydrate-containing food will reduce your risk of hypoglycaemia.

All alcoholic drinks are high in calories. Low-calorie mixers such as diet cola, diet ginger ale, diet tonic water help you to avoid extra calories.

Alcohol consumption is measured in units. One unit of alcohol is equal to half a pint of ordinary strength beer, lager, or cider or one pub measure (50ml) of sherry, vermouth, liqueur, or aperitif. There are 1.5 units of alcohol in one small glass (125ml) of wine or one pub measure (35ml) of spirits.

The maximum recommended daily intake of alcohol is one to two units for women and two to three for men. It is recommended that you have two alcohol-free days a week.

Why weight and body shape matter

Q What has my body shape got to do with diabetes?

If you carry extra fat around your waist rather than on your hips, you are at increased risk of developing heart and circulatory problems. Even if you are not overweight, your risk of heart disease is reduced if you have less fat around your waist than on your hips.

Q How do I know if I've got too much fat around my waist?

Measure your waist at the widest point. If it is more than 94cm (37in) for a man or 80cm (32in) for a woman, your risk of heart disease is increased.

Q How do I measure my waist-to-hip ratio?

Measure your waist and hips at the widest points and divide waist size by hip size. For example, a waist size of 82cm (33in) and hip size of 103cm (41in) gives a waist-to-hip ratio of 0.80. More than 0.95 (for a man) or 0.85 (for a woman) increases your risk of heart disease.

Q I thought that people with diabetes often lost weight before they were diagnosed. Is this a myth?

You can lose weight before you are diagnosed if your blood glucose level is very high. If your body cannot use glucose properly for energy, it starts to use fat stored in your muscles and under your skin. This happens more often at the onset of Type 1 diabetes because of the sudden shortage of insulin, and weight loss can be very rapid. With Type 2 diabetes, any weight loss would be more gradual (mainly due to not storing glucose efficiently and losing it in the urine). Your weight will be regained when blood glucose is more balanced.

Why are overweight and obese people more likely to develop Type 2 diabetes?

People who are overweight are much more likely to develop Type 2 diabetes because excess weight can make body cells resistant to the action of insulin. Although the pancreas still produces insulin, the body is unable to respond to it properly. In a person who doesn't have diabetes, insulin "unlocks" body cells and allows the uptake of glucose so that it can be used for fuel. However, in a person who has diabetes, insulin doesn't work properly and glucose stays in the bloodstream, raising the blood glucose level. See pp16–17 for an explanation of how diabetes affects blood glucose control.

How can losing weight help my diabetes?

Losing weight, even by a small amount, will make it easier to control your blood glucose level, lower your blood pressure and your cholesterol level, and prevent or delay the onset of other health problems, such as heart disease. Your body needs less insulin to process the glucose in your blood if your weight is in a normal range for your height. The insulin you produce also works better. Losing weight also means your heart and circulation work more efficiently.

How do I know if I am overweight?

You can tell if you are overweight by working out your body mass index (BMI; see p69) – this is considered the most standard way of assessing whether you are overweight. Your BMI is a ratio of your weight to your height. The figure that you come up with will tell you whether you are underweight, a healthy weight, overweight, or obese. If you have a body mass index of 25 or more, you are overweight. If you have a BMI of 30 or more, you are considered to be obese.

Q How do I work out my BMI?

You can work out your BMI by using a chart (see opposite) or you can calculate it on paper by dividing your weight in kilograms by the square of your height in metres. For example, if you weigh 70kg and your height is 1.67 metres, your BMI is 70 ÷ 2.79 (1.67 x 1.67) = 25.

Q I am overweight. Will losing weight mean that I can continue to manage my diabetes without tablets or insulin?

If you lose weight, you can reduce your body's need for insulin. This may prolong the time before you need to take tablets or insulin for your diabetes, although it is likely that you will still need to take medication at some point. Your health professional can help you to identify whether losing weight will achieve this for you or whether you need medication early, based on the test results of the blood glucose tests you do at home and your HbA1c test result (see pp113–114).

Q I am overweight. If I lose weight, will I be able to take a lower dose of tablets or insulin for my diabetes?

Possibly – it's likely that losing weight will enable the insulin you produce naturally to work better and this may mean that you can lower your dose of tablets or insulin – at the very least it will help your medication to work more effectively. Your health professional can discuss this with you.

Q Is it true that having diabetes can make me put on weight?

Type 2 diabetes on its own does not make you put on weight. However, there are other reasons why your weight may increase. Some of the tablets used to treat a high blood glucose level can cause weight gain or make it difficult for you to lose weight. Also, if you inject insulin this may cause you to gain some weight initially. Other causes of weight gain, such as eating too much for your level of activity, are not related to diabetes.

Working out your body mass index (BMI)

To find your BMI, measure your unclothed weight and your height. Trace a straight horizontal and vertical line from each measurement on the chart below. The point at which the two lines cross indicates the weight range you are in. You can then tell whether you need to gain weight, lose weight, or maintain your healthy weight.

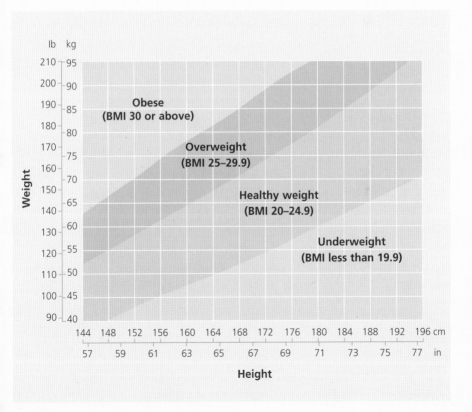

How to lose weight

Q I want to lose weight. Where do I start?

Eating fewer calories and burning more energy is the key to losing weight. This means eating healthily by cutting down on foods that are higher in fat and calories, and being more active in your daily life.

Q How much should I aim to lose a week?

Losing weight gradually is the most effective approach; "quick-fix" diets that lead to rapid weight loss are less healthy, and you are less likely to keep the weight off. Aiming to lose about 0.5–1kg (1–2lb) per week is a good starting point, although the exact amount will vary from one week to another. This is normal as you adjust to new patterns of eating and activity.

Q I've read that it's a good idea to keep a food diary. Why?

Keeping a food diary of what and when you eat and drink can make you aware of where you might be able to cut calories. It can also show you whether your meals are spread evenly throughout the day and whether snacking between meals is contributing to your weight.

Q How can a food diary help me to lose weight?

When you review your food diary, asking yourself the following questions can help you to identify where you can make changes: Do I eat high-fat or high-sugar foods at certain times of the day? Do I tend to sample food while I'm cooking? Do I use ordinary mixers with alcoholic drinks instead of diet versions? Do I dine out often? Do I eat very large meals? Analysing your answers to these questions may help you work out which changes will help you lose weight.

I've tried to lose weight in the past but usually give up after a week. How can I stay motivated?

Setting yourself small, short-term targets rather than long-term ones – for example, aiming to lose 1kg (2.2lb) by next week rather than 20kg (more than 3 stone) by next year – can make you more successful. Even if you lose only half a kilogram (1lb) in a week, as long as you are still following your eating and activity plan, your weight will continue to fall. Replacing tempting high-calorie foods in your fridge and cupboards with lower-calorie alternatives can help you stick to your plans. You may also find that recording your successes on a notice board together with inspirational pictures and encouraging notes helpful. Friends and family can help by being understanding about your aims.

A friend is trying to lose weight and she has written a detailed weight-loss plan. Should I be doing the same?

Yes – working through the following questions will help you come up with a plan. How much weight would you like to lose in the next few weeks? What changes are you going to make to what you eat and how much activity you do? How will you change your routine to fit these in? How will you measure your weight loss each week? How will you motivate yourself to achieve your weekly targets? Who will help you stay motivated? What will you do when you face obstacles? When will you start your plan? Is it realistic? If not, set yourself smaller targets that you will be able to achieve. Being successful once means you are likely to succeed again.

The last time I tried to eat less I ended up having hypos. How can I avoid this?

Testing your blood glucose level will let you know if your blood glucose is starting to drop and, if it is, reducing the dose of your tablets or insulin will compensate. Once you've lost weight, you are likely to need a lower dose of medication to prevent hypos.

Counting calories

Q How many calories should I cut out to lose weight?

To lose about 0.5kg (1lb) per week simply by eating less, you will need to reduce your calorie intake by 500 a day. To maintain this lower weight, women need to eat around 2,000 calories per day, men 2,500. Your health professional can help you to identify how changes to your calorie intake will affect your blood glucose level in order to help you avoid hypos.

Q How can I find out the calorie content of specific foods?

You may need to refer to a book listing the calorie content of foods, and weigh your food at first, to work out your calorie intake. Looking at food labels will also help you become familiar with energy values (see p53). A food diary can help you keep track of your calorie intake.

Q Is cutting down on fat the best way to reduce calories?

It is a good start. Fat is higher in calories than any type of food. Carbohydrate provides 3.75 calories per gram while fat provides 9 calories per gram – more than double the calories. Supermarkets offer low-fat options but often these are higher in sugar, so read the labels carefully.

Q Should I cut out carbohydrate or protein foods?

Even if you are eating less, you still need a variety of food types; excluding an entire food type, such as protein, is not healthy. Cutting out carbohydrate, your main energy source, is particularly unhealthy as your body will deplete its own energy stores to compensate.

Q What is meant by "hidden calories" in food?

Some foods can be deceiving. For example, biscuits are high in fat, as are some sauces that accompany meals; and alcohol contains a lot of calories.

How important is the size of the portions I eat at each meal? A large portion of lower-calorie food may contain the same number of calories as a small amount of high-fat food. If you enjoy eating larger portions, lower-calorie foods will suit you. If you still want to eat higher-fat foods, you may need to reduce your portion size.

CUTTING DOWN ON CALORIES

You can make simple choices on an everyday basis that will cut out calories and help you lose weight without denying yourself the foods you like. Below are some low-calorie alternatives to high-calorie foods and drinks.

HIGHER-CALORIE FOODS	CALS	LOWER-CALORIE ALTERNATIVE	CALS
100g carbonara sauce	200	100g tomato sauce	70
Small thick crust pizza	350	Small thin crust pizza	220
Medium bacon, lettuce, and tomato sandwich	502	Medium salmon and cucumber sandwich	274
300g can cream of tomato soup	216	300g can minestrone soup	93
Chicken breast with skin	300	Skinless chicken breast	190
50g cheddar cheese	215	50g cottage cheese	51
25g blue cheese dressing	115	25g low-fat Italian dressing	22
150g pot Greek yoghurt	195	150g pot low-fat yoghurt	80
40g salted peanuts	250	4 breadsticks	84
33ml can ordinary cola	135	330ml can diet cola	0
Small cappuccino	70	Regular-sized espresso	4

Q Is it safe to lose weight by missing a whole meal?

Eating regularly provides your body with the energy it needs and helps to keep your blood glucose in the recommended range. Skipping meals means you are likely to be hungrier by the time you do eat, and this may lead you to overeat and have an erratic blood glucose level.

Q If I eat more calories than I mean to, can I burn them off through physical activity?

Yes, although the exact amount of calories you burn depends on the intensity and duration of the activity you choose. Physical activity benefits you in two ways: it burns calories while you are doing the activity, and it raises your metabolic rate, which means that your body burns more calories even when you are resting.

Q If I eat the same number of calories but am more active, will I lose weight?

Whether you lose weight, or put it on, depends on how well your energy intake (in other words, calories) is matched to how much energy you use. You may find that if you are more active than you were in the past, you can lose some weight without altering your food intake. Whether you choose to count calories or not, your weight-loss plan will be more successful if you find a method that you are likely to be able to continue over the longer term.

Q Some diet plans suggest a number of portions of different types of foods. How does that relate to calories?

All eating plans to lose weight are based on a combination of food types and how many calories they contain. So a food plan based on portions means that the authors have already converted the calories for you, while trying to include foods that might help you feel less deprived. Choosing an eating plan that you can live with comfortably and therefore stick to in the long term is the most important factor for success.

Low calorie, low carbohydrate diets

I'm always reading about new weight-loss diets. Should I avoid them because I have diabetes?

It depends on the eating plan that is being recommended. The most effective ways to lose weight healthily are to reduce the number of calories that you eat and/or to burn calories through extra physical activity. Diets that provide extremely different amounts of the main food groups may not be suitable for you. If you think a particular eating plan might be for you, it may help to discuss it with your health professional.

Is it true that you can lose weight quickly by cutting out carbohydrates?

Diets such as the Atkin's diet work by forcing your body to burn fat and muscle for energy. This means that you can lose weight quickly but your body will replace the fat and muscle it has lost when you start eating normally again. This type of diet can be a "quick start" to losing weight, but cutting out carbohydrates means depriving your body of its main energy source.

Is it safe for me to follow a very low-carbohydrate diet?

If you take insulin or insulin-stimulating tablets, a very low-carbohydrate diet may cause hypos. Choosing healthy food options and generally reducing your calorie intake is the safest way to lose weight.

Can I replace one of my meals with a ready-made shake designed for slimmers?

Although ready-made shakes are designed to help you lose weight, you need to change your eating habits as well for a successful approach to weight loss. If you look at what foods you normally eat, then see where you can reduce excess calories, perhaps in discussion with your health professional, you can gradually adjust your food intake and maintain your lower weight.

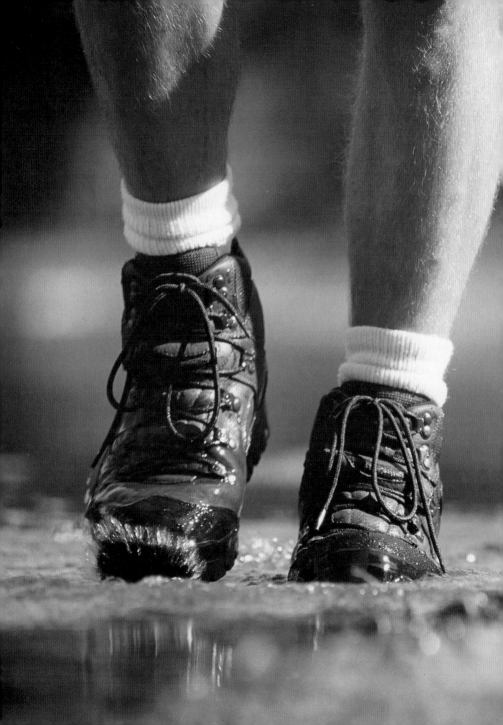

Physical activity

An active lifestyle helps your body to work more efficiently, benefiting both your general health and your diabetes. It can also help you to lose weight. Building more activity into your daily life is an important part of managing your diabetes.

The benefits of physical activity

Q I keep being told I should be more active – why?

Regular activity helps insulin you have produced or injected to work more efficiently. Being more active won't make your diabetes go away, but it can go a long way to helping you manage it. Another advantage is that it helps you to stay a healthy weight or lose weight if you need to.

Q How much physical activity do I need to do before I feel the benefits?

Any activity that raises your heart rate or makes you slightly out of breath will bring benefits. This doesn't necessarily mean joining a gym or doing strenuous activity. Activities such as dancing or walking briskly burn calories and help your circulation. The amount of activity to aim for is at least 30 minutes of moderate activity at least five times a week. This will help you to lose weight, regulate your blood glucose level, and reduce your risk of the long-term complications of diabetes.

Q How quickly can physical activity help me to lose weight?

If you combine regular physical activity with eating fewer calories, you may be able to lose half a kilogram (1–2lb) a week. Doing more physical activity can stimulate your appetite, so you may be tempted to eat high-calorie food if you feel hungry after activity. Snacking on low-calorie foods such as chopped raw vegetables or fruit will help you avoid too many calories. When you have lost weight, physical activity will help you maintain your new weight.

How does being more active help prevent the long-term complications of diabetes?

Regular physical activity helps insulin you have produced or injected to work more efficiently, which in turn contributes towards keeping your blood glucose and your blood pressure in the recommended ranges. These two benefits mean that you are less likely to develop the long-term complications of diabetes.

How will being active help my heart?

Regular activity helps to lower your blood pressure and your blood cholesterol levels, which means that you have less chance of having a heart attack or a stroke. It also makes your heart stronger and more efficient so that it can pump more blood with every heartbeat, and it reduces your risk of having a heart attack from clots forming in your coronary arteries. The more active you are, the less likely you are to have a heart attack, and the greater your chance of surviving a heart attack if you were to have one.

I'm prone to depression. Will being active help me?

Yes, activity raises your levels of endorphins and serotonin. These brain chemicals influence your mood and sense of wellbeing and have a strong antidepressant effect. Some types of activity, for example, playing golf or tennis also mean spending time with other people, and this can help to lift your spirits, too.

I don't take tablets or insulin yet. Will staying active allow me to carry on without medication?

The progressive nature of diabetes means you will probably need tablets or insulin eventually, but with an active lifestyle, you may delay the need for medication because regular activity reduces your insulin resistance. Activity can help at any stage. If you already take tablets, increasing your activity levels may help to delay the need to start injecting insulin and reduce the dose you need.

Myth "You have to spend a lot of time being active to get any benefit"

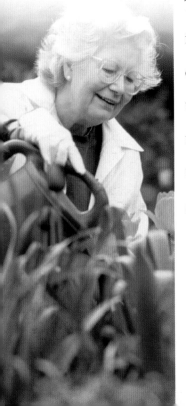

Truth The recommended amount of activity is 30 minutes at least five times a week. But you don't necessarily have to dedicate specific times to this – you can feel the benefits just by being more active in your day-to-day life. Everyday things such as climbing stairs, going shopping, gardening, and housework all count as activity.

Will I still need to take my diabetes medication if I become more active?

Yes, but you may need a lower dose to achieve the same effect. If you are on insulin-stimulating tablets, you may be more at risk of a hypo when you become more active, so you may need a reduction in the dose of your tablets or a change to a different type of tablet. Also, if you are more active, you may find you lose weight. If you lose more than a few kilograms you are likely to need a lower dose of tablets or insulin.

I've been told I have impaired glucose tolerance. Will being more physically active help me?

Yes, having impaired glucose tolerance means that you are more likely to go on to develop Type 2 diabetes. Becoming more active, especially if you also lose weight, will help your natural insulin to work as effectively as possible to regulate your blood glucose level. Once you have impaired glucose tolerance, you will always be at risk of developing diabetes, but the more active you are, the longer it may take to develop.

I'm 65 this year, isn't it a bit late to start being more active?

It's never too late to become more active. You don't have to start a vigorous or ambitious form of activity – just becoming more active generally throughout your day (see pp88–89) will help your blood glucose level and blood pressure to stay in the recommended ranges. Being active will also help you to feel more energetic over time.

How is physical activity beneficial after a heart attack?

Regular activity will help to strengthen your blood vessels and improve blood circulation to your heart. Physical activity can also help to prevent stress, depression, and anxiety after you have had a heart attack, and this can go a long way to helping you to recover and feel like your usual self again.

Physical activity and your blood glucose level

Q What happens to my blood glucose level when I'm active?

Gentle activity for 10–30 minutes is unlikely to have much effect on your blood glucose level. However, more vigorous activity will cause your blood glucose level to fall because of the extra glucose your muscles are using. When you stop activity, your muscles and, to a lesser extent, your liver, replace their glycogen stores by taking glucose from your bloodstream. The longer or more intense the activity, the more glucose you need to replenish these stores, so your blood glucose level could be affected for several hours.

Q Can a lot of physical activity cause a hypo?

If you take insulin-stimulating tablets or insulin, physical activity can sometimes cause your blood glucose level to fall below 4 millimoles per litre so that you have a hypo either at the time or some hours later. This is more likely if an activity is intense or prolonged. It's important to understand what effect particular activities have on your blood glucose level so that you can take action to prevent or treat a hypo if you need to.

Q My blood glucose drops when I mow the lawn. What can I do to prevent this?

If your blood glucose level is 5 millimoles per litre or lower before gardening, eating a snack such as fruit will raise your blood glucose level and reduce your risk of a hypo. Another option is reducing your medication before you mow. If your level is higher beforehand, you may not need to snack or reduce your medication.

Why did I feel anxious and shaky during a recent shopping trip?

Shopping is a physical activity and may have caused your blood glucose level to fall. If you take insulin or insulin-stimulating tablets, walking in and out of shops, climbing stairs, and carrying heavy bags can increase your risk of a hypo.

How will I know the effect of activity on my blood glucose?

Testing your blood glucose level before and after activity, and again a few hours later will tell you. If you are active for more than an hour, check your blood glucose level in the middle of the activity to help you find out if you need to take action to prevent a hypo.

THE IMPACT OF ACTIVITY ON BLOOD GLUCOSE

If you are moderately active for 30 minutes or more, your blood glucose level changes throughout the activity. The more intense or long-lasting the activity, the greater the impact on your blood glucose. Knowing the effect of your activity can help you decide how to manage your diabetes.

DURATION OF ACTIVITY	EFFECT ON BLOOD GLUCOSE
Approx 0–15 minutes	Blood glucose level rises slightly as your body converts glycogen stored in your liver into glucose in your blood.
Approx 15–30 minutes	Blood glucose level falls slightly as your muscles start to use up the glucose available in your body.
Approx 30–45 minutes	Blood glucose level could fall even further as more glucose is used up by your muscles to keep them working.
End of activity	Blood glucose level continues to fall as your liver and muscles replace their glycogen stores by taking glucose from your bloodstream.

Q Can strenuous activity in the day cause a hypo in the night?

Yes, your blood glucose level can sometimes take up to 36 hours to return to normal after strenuous activity. This is because your body is gradually replacing the stores of glucose in your muscles. It is important to test your blood glucose level before you go to bed so that you can take any necessary action to reduce the chances of a hypo during the night.

Q Does having sex make a difference to my blood glucose level?

Yes, sex is an activity like any other. If you have very active sex or sex that goes on for a long time, your blood glucose level is likely to fall. Testing your blood glucose level before and after sex will help you identify if you need to take action to avoid having a hypo.

Q Being more active doesn't seem to make any difference to my blood glucose level. Why?

The intensity or duration of your activity may not be enough to affect your blood glucose level. Alternatively, if your blood glucose level is raised before your activity, and it doesn't fall as you expect, you may not have enough insulin to help your muscles use the extra glucose your body is producing. In this case, you may need to increase your tablets or insulin dose – talking with your health professional can help you decide.

Q Can I make adjustments to the dose of my tablets or insulin before physical activity?

Yes, if you know in advance that an activity will make your blood glucose level fall, you can reduce your dose of tablets or insulin beforehand. If your activity is unplanned, or you know that it won't make a major difference to your blood glucose level, you could have a small snack beforehand instead. Checking your blood glucose level after physical activity will help you to identify whether you need to eat a carbohydrate snack to prevent it dropping too low.

EATING TO CONTROL YOUR BLOOD GLUCOSE LEVEL BEFORE ACTIVITY

If you take insulin or insulin-stimulating tablets and prefer not to reduce your dose before you are active, this information will help you decide what snacks to eat. This is based on the intensity and duration of the activity you do, together with your pre-activity blood glucose level in millimoles per litre.

TYPE AND DURATION OF ACTIVITY	BLOOD GLUCOSE BEFORE ACTIVITY	EXAMPLES OF WHAT TO EAT 30 MINUTES BEFORE ACTIVITY
Gentle For example, walking or cycling for less than 30 minutes.	5 or less	One slice of bread or one piece of fruit.
	Any level above 5	No carbohydrate needed.
Moderate For example, playing golf, brisk walking, dancing, or swimming for 1 hour.	5 or less	One slice of bread plus one piece of fruit.
	5–9	One slice of bread plus one piece of fruit.
	9–13	No carbohydrate needed.
	Above 13	Activity not advised until your blood glucose level is lower.
Intense For example, playing football or tennis for 2 hours. Vigorously cycling or swimming for more than 1 hour.	5 or less	Two slices of bread plus one piece of fruit.
	5–9	One slice of bread plus one piece of fruit.
	9–13	One slice of bread or one piece of fruit.
	Above 13	Activity not advised until your blood glucose level is lower.

Incorporating activity into your life

Q Can I do anything to become more physically active at home?

Yes, vigorous housework, gardening, and walking up and down stairs more often are activities that keep you moving and increase your heart rate. You might also want to use demonstration videos or DVDs at home.

Q Is it worth buying exercise equipment to use at home?

Good quality equipment is expensive and can take up a fair amount of space in your home. Thinking about whether you will use it on a long-term basis will help you decide if it is worth purchasing.

Q What type of equipment can I buy?

There is a huge range of exercise equipment available, but before you buy you can try out different machines in a gym to see which ones you enjoy using. Popular pieces of equipment include exercise bikes, treadmills, rowing machines, and step machines. Some have extra features, such as a variety of programmes and a built-in heart rate monitor, for example.

Q I've got a hectic work schedule. How can I fit physical activity into my routine?

It can be helpful to identify times in your working day when you could set aside 10–30 minutes to be active. For example, walking part or all of the way to or from work, or going for a walk at lunchtime. If you have a desk job it is even more important to consider ways to keep active. Getting up from your desk and moving around whenever you can, and using the stairs in preference to the lift might be options for you.

I'm worried I might need to spend a lot of time doing an activity to get the benefits – is this true?

You don't necessarily have to dedicate specific times to being active – you might be able to introduce more activity into your day by staying on the move, walking briskly, cycling instead of driving a car, getting off the bus a stop early, and avoiding prolonged periods of sitting down. The recommended amount of activity is 30 minutes at least five times a week, but you'll also feel the benefits if you are generally more active every day.

I'm now more active throughout the day. How can I measure my progress?

Losing weight, lower blood glucose and blood pressure levels, and feeling fitter are all measures of progress. You may want to use an electronic device to measure these effects. For example, you could measure your heartbeat with a heart rate monitor, which consists of a strap that you wear around your chest and a watch device. Or you could wear a pedometer, which counts how many steps you take in a day.

Does having diabetes mean that I should avoid some physical activities?

Having diabetes places no restrictions on the type of physical activity you can do. But as with everyone, building up your fitness gradually is recommended. If you want to increase your muscle bulk or train for an endurance sport, your programme can be tailored to your needs. The chart on p94 gives more information on the fitness benefits of different activities.

I had a heart attack last year. Should I avoid exertion?

Physical activity is particularly important if you already have heart problems, but consulting your health professional before embarking on an activity programme will help you to plan what you do. Starting slowly and increasing your activity very gradually are likely to be recommended.

Getting started and keeping going

Q I've been inactive for so long. Where do I start?

If you haven't been active for some time, it's sensible to start with a gentle activity, such as walking, swimming, or simply becoming more active around the house. You can build on this gradually over time – see pp92–95. If you take insulin-stimulating tablets or insulin, measuring your blood glucose level before and after any new activity will help you assess its impact – if your blood glucose level falls below 4 millimoles per litre, you will need to treat yourself for a hypo (see p128).

Q How can I find out how fit (or unfit) I am?

If you are unable to climb one or two flights of stairs without being short of breath, or if you are unable to carry on a conversation when you are walking briskly, this suggests you could benefit from being more active. Being fitter means you can do 30 minutes of moderate physical activity, making you sweat and breathe harder, at least five times a week.

Q How should I warm up and cool down?

If your chosen activity is fairly intense, it is important to warm up your muscles so that they work better and are less prone to injury. You can do this by doing your chosen activity at a slow pace for the first 10 minutes. Afterwards, cool down by decreasing the intensity of the exercise for the last 10 minutes. Finish by gently stretching your arms, legs, and back muscles – this will help to prevent you becoming stiff or injured.

My health professional suggested I work out an activity plan. Why?

Creating an activity plan (see pp96–97) will help to give you a clear idea of your goals and how you are going to achieve them. Long-term changes in your approach to physical activity will give you the most benefit, so it makes good sense to look at your overall activity from the start.

How do I know if I'm being active enough?

Feeling warmer and slightly out of breath are signs of your activity being effective. If you can sing while you are active, you could probably work harder; if you feel you are gasping for breath, you are probably doing too much too quickly. You should not exercise so hard that you experience pain, and you should stop if you feel nauseous, dizzy, or unwell.

I don't always feel like being active although I know I'm meant to. How can I get motivated?

An activity plan (see pp96–97) that specifies realistic daily goals can be a great source of motivation. Putting your plan in a prominent place will act as a reminder, and recording any achievements in terms of weight loss, improved blood glucose levels, or simply feeling better or fitter will help motivate you. You may find a reward each time you reach a specific milestone can also help. If you feel you will be encouraged by being active with other people, you might like to try joining an exercise class or a walking group, or arrange to do an activity with a friend or partner.

I used to swim a lot but then I got ill and stopped. How can I get started again?

Your activity level may take time to build up again. Developing a new activity plan and working out what type and intensity of activity is right for you now will help you to get back to being active and swimming as soon as you can.

Becoming more active

Whatever your circumstances or lifestyle, you can become more active. The goal to work towards is a total of 30 minutes of activity at least five times a week. This doesn't have to be 30 minutes of continuous activity. You might want to break it down into three sets of 10 minutes, for example. A good way of measuring how active you are is to see how many steps you take over the course of a day, using a device known as a pedometer. Your aim should be to build up to 10,000 steps a day. As you gradually become more active, building in rewards for your achievements can help you to stay motivated.

HOW FIT ARE YOU?

It is a good idea to assess your level of fitness before you start any regular activity. You may be surprised at the amount of activity you already do, or you may feel that you want to do more. You can assess your fitness by answering the following questions:

• Can you climb one or two flights of stairs without being short of breath or feeling heaviness or tiredness in your legs?

• Do you normally take the stairs rather than the escalator or lift?

• Are you able to maintain a conversation during light to moderate activity such as walking?

• Would you walk a 10-minute journey rather than take the car?

• Do you do 30 minutes of moderate activity that makes you feel warmer and breathe harder at least five times a week?

If you answered "no" to any of the questions above, you could benefit from fitting more activity into your daily routine.

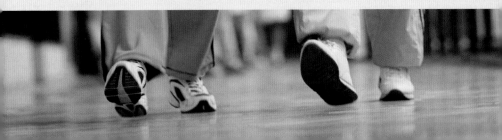

INCREASING YOUR LEVEL OF ACTIVITY

Before starting on any new activity, you may want to consult your health professional first. If you have been very inactive, start slowly. For example, if you want to start running, begin by walking more and jogging for short spells between walking.

IF YOU ARE VERY INACTIVE

Try starting with simple extra movements, such as manually changing the channel on the TV rather than using the remote control, leaving the phone away from you so that you have to move to answer it, or walking round the room before sitting down. You could gradually increase the number of times you do these activities, and set yourself targets, such as not sitting down for more than an hour at a time.

IF YOU ARE MODERATELY ACTIVE

Try to build upon the amount of activity you already do by, for example, adding an extra 5–10 minutes to your walk, cycle ride, gardening session, or swim. Or increase the intensity of an activity. Set yourself a longer-term goal, such as a 5-mile walk in a month's time, training for a charity swim, or joining an aerobics class.

IF YOU ARE REGULARLY ACTIVE

The most important thing is to stay motivated by keeping activities varied, doing activities with family or friends, or linking activity with a reward: a brisk walk to see a friend, a cycle-ride ending in a drink or meal, or a hot bath after the gym.

CALORIES BURNED BY ACTIVITIES

Activity	Calories per 30 mins
Climbing stairs	**330**
Gardening, digging	**240**
Mowing the lawn	**140**
House cleaning	**120**
Shopping	**120**
Gardening, weeding	**105**
Ironing	**60**

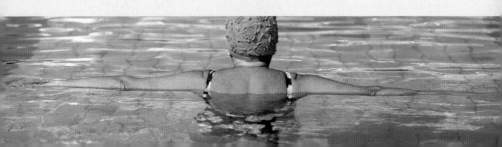

Choosing a physical activity

Q What is the best type of activity to help me lose weight?

Aerobic activities are the best way to burn calories and lose weight. This includes anything that raises your heart rate and makes you breathe faster. Activities such as walking, gardening, cleaning, and climbing stairs are all aerobic activities; so too are dancing, swimming, cycling, and aerobics classes. The more aerobic activity you do, and the longer you do it for, the more calories you will burn.

Q I get out of breath when I walk upstairs. What can I do to develop more stamina?

Increasing your activity level gradually is a good way to develop your stamina. For example, trying to be a little more active by going for a 10-minute walk or gardening for a little longer than usual, or doing extra housework, will all build stamina. As you become fitter, you will soon notice that you can keep going for longer and are less likely to be breathless after minor exertion. Monitoring your fitness level by keeping a record of your progress may motivate you to stay active.

Q What type of activity is good for stress relief?

Almost any type of activity is good for combating stress because activity causes the release of brain chemicals known as endorphins and serotonin, which have a positive effect on your mood and sense of wellbeing. You might find that taking part in gentle, non-competitive, or meditative activities such as yoga, t'ai chi, or swimming helps you to deal with stress.

What physical activities can I do with my partner?

Finding activities you both enjoy will make it easier to keep motivated. Walking, cycling, or hiking together, playing badminton or tennis either indoors or outdoors, or going to dancing classes together, might all be options for you.

I enjoy physical activity with a group but don't want to go to an aerobics class. What else can I do?

Other group activities include joining a rambling group, playing golf, cricket, or bowls or going to a stretching or yoga class. You might like to try aqua-aerobics, which is a more gentle and low-impact alternative to conventional aerobics.

I have high blood pressure. Are there any activities that I should avoid?

If you have high blood pressure, becoming or staying physically active is very important. The only activities to avoid are weight-lifting, and sports such as squash, which are quite vigorous and demand intense activity. If you are very overweight, have heart or breathing problems, have been inactive for a long time, or your blood pressure is very high, talking with your health professional before you take up a new activity will help you get started safely. Relaxation exercises can be helpful if you have high blood pressure.

How can I find a physical activity that I enjoy?

A good starting point for creating your activity plan (see pp96–97) is to think about activities you have enjoyed in the past. Is activity a way of getting some time to yourself, or is it a way to meet people and be sociable? Do you enjoy being outdoors or indoors? Do you like being at home or going out? Do you enjoy competing with others, either individually or in teams? The answers to these questions will guide you towards an activity that you will enjoy.

Q How can I best take care of myself while being physically active?

Drinking plenty of water to avoid becoming dehydrated will help. Monitoring the effect of your activity on your blood glucose by testing frequently and taking action to avoid a hypo if you need to will help keep your blood glucose well balanced. Talking with your health professional will give you specific information about an activity programme that will fit in with your diabetes.

FITNESS BENEFITS OF DIFFERENT ACTIVITIES

When selecting a new activity, you can choose which aspect of your health and fitness to work upon: weight loss, stamina, flexibility, or strength. The fitness benefits of some suggested forms of activity are shown below. One square indicates a small benefit; four squares indicates a major benefit.

ACTIVITY	CALS PER 30 MINS	STAMINA	FLEXIBILITY	STRENGTH
Aerobics	215	■■■■	■■■	■■
Cycling (fast)	280	■■■■	■■■	■■■
Golf	195	■	■■	■■
Hiking	200	■■■	■	■■
Jogging	245	■■■■	■■	■■
Swimming (fast)	300	■■■■	■■■■	■■■■
Tennis	210	■■	■■■	■■■
Walking (brisk)	180	■■■■	■■■	■■
Aqua-aerobics	140	■	■■■■	■
Yoga	135	■	■■■■	■

My health professional told me that I should look after my feet more when I go hiking. Why?

Long periods of walking can make you vulnerable to foot injuries. For example, a stone in your shoe or friction from a shoe or boot can lead to cuts, blisters, and inflammation. If you have reduced blood flow or nerve damage to your feet, you may not be able to feel this kind of damage and it may quickly become worse. This means that minor foot problems can develop into ulcers. Making sure that your socks and hiking shoes or boots fit your feet perfectly and don't rub will help prevent this.

Should I avoid rambling and jogging if I have blisters on my feet?

Yes, waiting until the blisters on your feet have completely healed will ensure that they do not become worse or infected through added pressure or rubbing. See pp135–137 for more information about caring for your feet.

My 16-year-old son has Type 2 diabetes and is very inactive. What activities could he do?

If your son is overweight, he may not feel confident about participating in team sports, but he might be happier doing other types of activity. For example, if he frequently travels short distances by car or public transport, he could start walking or cycling instead. At home, he could help you with DIY jobs, washing the car, or mowing the lawn – offering him a reward might act as an extra incentive for doing these things. You might also want to lead by example by becoming more active yourself or as a family, with trips to your leisure centre or walking in the park. As your son becomes fitter and loses weight, he may feel more confident and want to take up an activity that he has expressed an interest in – such as skateboarding, working out in the gym, or football.

Making activity work for you

You might have ambitious plans when it comes to physical activity, but if an activity is difficult to fit into your lifestyle or you don't enjoy it very much, you may find it difficult to stay motivated. You are more likely to be successful if you spend some time working through the points below and create your own unique activity plan to match your needs and lifestyle.

MAKING AN ACTIVITY PLAN

① WHAT ARE YOUR GOALS?

Deciding what you want to achieve – for example relaxation, feeling fitter, losing weight, or lowering your blood pressure or cholesterol level – will help you identify the activity that's right for you.

② WHICH ACTIVITY?

Choosing activities that you like and that you can achieve will help you to plan realistically. Use the tips opposite to think about what you'd like to do. Remember it's never too late to start something new as long as you start gently and gradually.

③ WHEN CAN YOU BE MORE ACTIVE?

Identifying the time you have available, whether it is part of your usual day or if you need to put time aside, will help you to plan. You may need to do this each week if your lifestyle is very variable.

④ WHAT WILL GET IN THE WAY?

Planning your time around other commitments you have will increase your chance of success. Thinking of ways to avoid potential distractions will also help.

⑤ WRITE DOWN YOUR PLAN

A written plan can help you to remember your goals and help you to record what you are achieving. See opposite for an example of an activity plan for one week.

⑥ ASSESS YOUR PLAN

At the end of each week, assess how well you've done. Do you need to make any changes your activity plan? For example, if you have achieved all your goals, you might want to do more next week. If too many things got in the way, giving yourself a more realistic plan, for example smaller goals, might help.

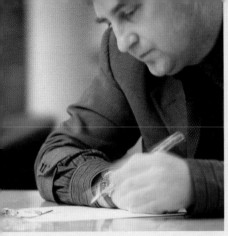

CHOOSING YOUR ACTIVITY

Different activities have different benefits. The following tips may help you think about new activities and making a choice that works best for you.

- Jogging, cycling, hiking, and going to the gym can help you lose weight and lower your blood pressure and blood fats.
- Gentle stretching, t'ai chi, and swimming can help you to relax and unwind.
- Yoga and Pilates can improve your muscle strength and posture.
- Running up stairs, cycling instead of driving, and walking during work breaks can help you fit activity into a busy day.
- Using an exercise bike or video at home are useful if you prefer to be active alone.
- Rambling with a group, golf, tennis, and playing bowls are ways of combining activity with socialising.

SAMPLE ACTIVITY PLAN

MONDAY
10-minute walk immediately after breakfast with my wife
10-minute walk to visit my friend in the evening

TUESDAY
20 minutes weeding in the garden

WEDNESDAY
15 minutes on my exercise bike after work

THURSDAY
Long day at work – no extra activity

FRIDAY
Walk to the local shops – 15 minutes each way

SATURDAY
Wash my car by hand in the afternoon

SUNDAY
Clean the kitchen floor
Play tennis with my wife (first time!)

Short-term goals (over next 3 weeks):
Go swimming on Monday and Thursday evenings for 30 minutes at a time.
Walk rather than drive to the shops on Tuesday and Friday.

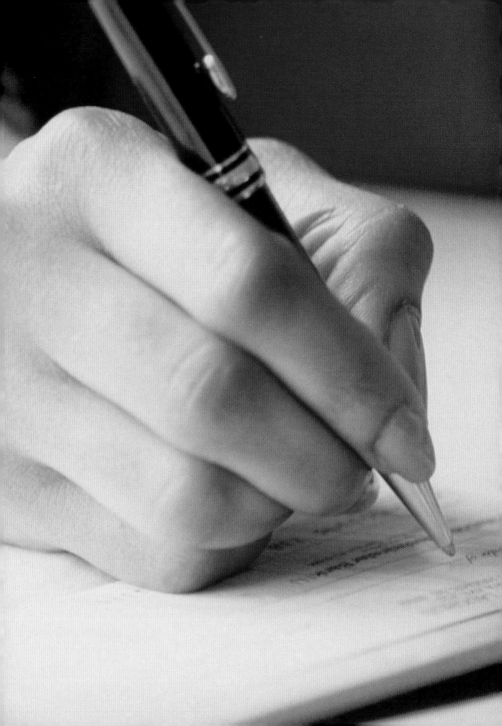

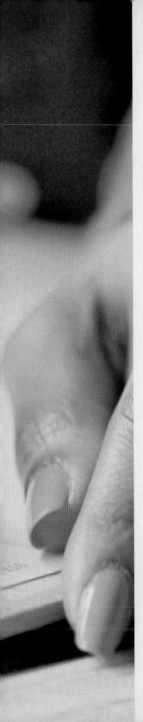

Monitoring your diabetes

Monitoring the amount of glucose in your blood is part of your daily diabetes care. It helps you identify any adjustments to your treatment or lifestyle that might be necessary. Your blood pressure and blood fat levels, which are likely to be raised, also need to be monitored regularly.

Understanding your blood glucose level

Q Why do I need to monitor my blood glucose level?

The only way to know if your blood glucose level is within the recommended range is to take a sample of your blood and measure the amount of glucose in it. This is important even if you are eating healthily and being active. Regular tests tell you how your blood glucose level is affected by your food, the amount and type of activity you do, and by the impact of stress and illness. If your blood glucose level is regularly too high you are more likely to develop long-term complications.

Q What level of blood glucose should I be aiming for?

Blood glucose is measured in millimoles per litre. The ideal range is 4–7 millimoles per litre. Even when your blood glucose is well controlled, you are always likely to get occasional results outside of this range, but it is the general pattern of your results that is important.

Q Why can't I rely on symptoms to tell me whether my blood glucose level is too high or low?

If your blood glucose is slightly raised (between 7–10 millimoles per litre), you probably won't have symptoms (your body only starts producing larger amounts of urine when your blood glucose is above this level). If you regularly have high readings, you may not get symptoms until your blood glucose level is 15 millimoles per litre or higher. With a low blood glucose level, it can be dangerous to wait for symptoms, because by this point you may be feeling too confused or disorientated to treat yourself.

What should I do if I keep getting high blood glucose levels?

These levels might be caused by you gaining weight, eating more, or being less active than usual. If you know that one of these factors is responsible, you may be able to remedy it yourself. If you still have high readings for no obvious reason over a week or two, you may need to alter your medication. Your health professional can help you to identify what changes you might need to make.

I often get readings below 4 millimoles per litre, but feel fine. Am I hypo or not?

Yes, a "hypo" means any blood glucose level below 4 millimoles per litre, although the level at which you start to have symptoms may vary. If you have had diabetes for years and have often had hypos, your body may no longer give you any early warning symptoms. Keeping your blood glucose level above 4 millimoles per litre and taking glucose whenever it drops lower will help to restore your early warning symptoms.

I'm taking insulin and sometimes I have a hypo and then a very high reading later. Why does this happen?

If you have readings below 4 millimoles per litre, your body will produce extra glucose to help you recover, which contributes to the high reading a few hours later. Preventing the hypos, either by reducing your insulin dose or making other changes, will help prevent the high readings that follow.

My uncle has diabetes and tests his urine for glucose. Why have I been taught to test my blood?

Urine testing was once the standard way to monitor diabetes, but it is not accurate as it will show a positive result only when your blood glucose is around 10 millimoles per litre or above. Blood testing is more accurate and up-to-date. Your uncle could discuss with his health professional whether it would be helpful for him to test his blood instead.

Q How frequently should I check my blood glucose level?

This will depend on what information you need at the time. For example, if your medication has changed or if you are ill, you may need a lot of information and be testing 4–7 times a day. At times when your blood glucose level does not vary much, you might test a lot less frequently than this and, on some days, you may not test at all. Your health professional can help you work out how often you should test. The main reason for testing is to find out what action you need to take to keep your blood glucose in the recommended range.

FACTORS THAT AFFECT YOUR BLOOD GLUCOSE

These everyday factors have an influence on your blood glucose level. Understanding the effect of each will mean you can take action to prevent your blood glucose level rising too high or falling too low.

FACTOR	EFFECT
Carbohydrate foods	Raise your blood glucose. How quickly and how much depends on the type and quantity.
Physical activity	Lowers your blood glucose by helping insulin to work more efficiently and using up energy.
Insulin injections	Lower your blood glucose. How quickly and for how long depends on the type of insulin.
Diabetes tablets	Lower your blood glucose.
Stress	Likely to raise your blood glucose; rarely, may lower it.
Illness	Raises your blood glucose.

At what times of day should I check my blood glucose?

Testing before a meal tells you what your blood glucose level is when it is least affected by food. Also, testing 2 hours after a meal tells you how well your body has used the glucose from your meal. Testing before you go to bed will tell you whether you need to take any action to keep your blood glucose in the recommended range during the night. Testing at one or more of these times helps you to build up a picture of what happens to your blood glucose level at different times of the day and in response to food and medication. You may want to test at other times, for example, if you want to find out the effect of physical activity on your blood glucose level.

In what situations is it really important for me to test?

If you inject insulin or take insulin-stimulating tablets, testing your blood glucose level if you start to feel "hypo" helps you take action quickly. Testing your blood glucose level before you drive and taking action if you need to will help you avoid a hypo while driving. Testing when you are ill is also important.

When might I need to check my blood glucose level more frequently than usual?

You may want to test more often when your diabetes treatment changes or if you are diagnosed with long-term complications such as kidney or eye problems. There are also short-term situations in which you might need more information about your blood glucose level: for example, when you are ill, when you are drinking alcohol, and when you are in a hot climate. Also, if your weight changes, you become more or less active, or your eating patterns change, testing more often can help you check that your blood glucose level is still in the recommended range. If it isn't, you can take steps to remedy it before it starts to cause longer-term damage.

Monitoring equipment

Specialized equipment is available for you to test your blood glucose level wherever you are. Testing is usually done by inserting a blood testing strip into a blood glucose meter and applying a blood sample (obtained using a lancet) to the testing strip to obtain a reading. Your health professional can help you decide what type of equipment is best for you. You can also get information from books, the internet, or Diabetes UK (a national diabetes organization, see p200). Testing strips and lancets are obtained on prescription. You can buy meters from a pharmacy or your health professional may give you a starter kit.

BLOOD GLUCOSE METERS

Battery-operated devices called glucose meters analyse the amount of glucose in the blood sample on your testing strip and then display the result on a screen. With most meters, you insert a testing strip into the meter before applying your blood to a specific area on the strip. The meters use one of two different methods to analyse the results but both are highly accurate and give results ranging from 0.6–33.3 millimoles per litre. Some meters also have additional features – for example, one type includes its own lancing device for collecting a blood sample.

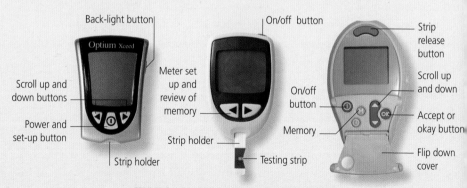

SELECTION OF STANDARD BLOOD GLUCOSE METERS

LANCING DEVICES AND BLOOD GLUCOSE STRIPS

Most lancing devices consist of a hand-held tube into which you put a needle (lancet). A dial enables you to choose how deeply the needle enters your site. Lancets are used with a lancing device to prick your skin. They are designed to be used once to avoid infection and to make sure the needle is as sharp as possible. Blood testing strips usually come in packs of 25 or 50. Always check the expiry date of your blood testing strips before use.

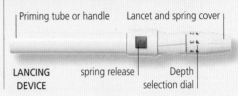

Priming tube or handle   Lancet and spring cover

LANCING   spring release   Depth
DEVICE   selection dial

CHOOSING A METER

Considering the following factors will help you to choose a glucose meter.

Size Some meters are smaller and more compact than others. If you have problems with dexterity, you may find a larger meter helpful.

Result display Meters with large displays may be easier to read if you have vision problems. Some meters just give you your test result, others give the date and time.

Averages Many meters provide you with an average of your readings, for example, over the previous 7, 14, or 28 days.

Computer download facility Some meters have a facility that allows you to download your results and analyse them on a computer.

Size of blood sample The amount of blood you need to put on your strip can vary from 0.3 to 10 microlitres.

Memory Meters vary greatly in the number of results they can store. Some can store 10; others can store up to 450. A large memory is useful if you aren't always able to write down your results.

Timing After you have applied blood, meters can take anything from 5–45 seconds to give you a result.

Testing sites All meters can analyse blood from your fingertips. Some can also analyse blood from your forearm, the palm of your hand, or your abdomen.

Additional features Some devices combine a blood glucose meter with other features, such as a lancing device.

Carrying out a blood glucose test

Q Do blood glucose meters all work in the same way?

No. The exact procedure for carrying out a blood test will vary according to which type of blood glucose meter you have. With most machines, you will need to prepare the meter for use (see opposite), insert a blood testing strip, obtain a blood sample, apply blood to the testing strip, and wait for a result. Checking the instructions that come with your meter will help you identify any variations to this routine.

Q How can I ensure I get the most accurate result possible?

Your blood glucose meter will come with instructions on how to use it, so the first step is to read and follow these. The following additional tips should also help to make sure the reading you get is accurate: wash and dry the site you intend to take blood from; calibrate your meter each time you start a new pot of testing strips; use a new testing strip for each test. Also, avoid "topping up" blood on your strip if your equipment isn't designed for this.

Q Why does my blood glucose meter turn itself off before I've done a test?

If you insert your testing strip into the meter and then take too long to apply your blood, your meter switches itself off to save battery power. If this happens, you need to remove the testing strip and reinsert it. Once you have put a drop of blood on the testing strip and the strip is in the meter, an in-built timing device takes over.

PREPARING A BLOOD GLUCOSE METER FOR USE

Blood testing strips vary from batch to batch (they may contain different amounts of chemicals), so you need to calibrate most meters every time you start a new pack of strips to obtain an accurate result. Testing your meter at least once a month with a quality control solution (which contains a known amount of glucose) will enable you to check your machine is measuring blood glucose correctly.

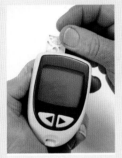

① If your meter has a coding chip provided with the strips, insert the chip into the slot on the meter. If it has a coding strip, insert this into the meter, then remove it once the code has been registered. If it has a code (C) button, insert the strip, then press the button until the code matches the one on the new pack of strips.

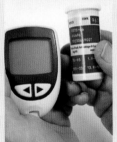

② When you insert a test strip, compare the code number on the display with the number printed on the test strip container. The two numbers must be identical. If they are not identical, repeat the above coding procedure until the correct code number is displayed.

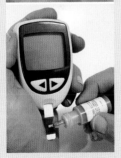

③ To test using the quality control solution, apply the solution to the test strip in the same way as you would apply your blood, then compare the control solution result with the range printed on the test strip or control solution packet. The result will fall within this range if your meter is reading accurately.

OBTAINING A BLOOD SAMPLE

Blood tests form part of your day-to-day routine when you have diabetes. Although your finger is the most common site to use, you can also test blood from your forearm, the palm of your hand, or your abdomen – if your equipment is designed to test blood from these sites. Following these steps will help to ensure that you get an accurate reading from your blood glucose test.

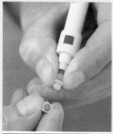

① Wash your hands and then rub them to increase your circulation. Put a fresh lancet into your lancing device and remove its disposable cap. Replace the lancing device's cover and turn the dial to set your preferred depth level. Switch on your blood glucose meter, or insert the test strip into your meter to switch it on.

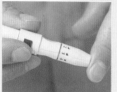

② Put your lancing device firmly against the side of the tip of your finger. Press the button on the side or end of the device to fire the lancet. Move the lancing device away from your finger and wait a few seconds for the blood to flow.

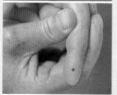

③ If a drop of blood doesn't appear, apply pressure to the base of your finger to assist your blood flow. If you still can't get enough blood, start again using another finger and a new test strip, and increase the depth setting if necessary.

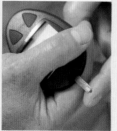

④ When you have enough blood, apply it to the pad on the end of the testing strip. Depending on the type of strip, wait 5–45 seconds for your meter to display your blood glucose level. Dispose of your lancet and strip in a recommended sharps box.

Is there a device that can continuously monitor my blood glucose level?

There are two types of device available for continuous testing: a watch-like device that you wear on your wrist and a machine that is connected to a needle in your abdomen. These are not widely used, partly because they are more expensive than a blood glucose meter and partly because the technology is still being developed. If you use this equipment, you still need to do some fingerprick tests to calibrate the machines, and you need to buy ongoing supplies for the equipment.

Why do I need to keep a diary of my test results?

Recording the results of your blood glucose tests will enable you to see how your blood glucose level changes over the course of a day or a week. If you notice patterns of high and low blood glucose readings, you can take action to bring your blood glucose level back within the recommended range.

What information do I need to put in my monitoring diary?

A monitoring diary provides space for you to enter the results of seven or more blood glucose tests a day, together with the date and time of the tests. You can also record what type and dose of medication you are taking plus any additional relevant information, such as what has caused high or low readings or what changes you are making to correct fluctuating readings.

Can I create an electronic diary?

Yes, some blood glucose meters have a facility that allows you to download your results and analyse them on a computer. This facility enables you to view your results in graph or table form, and you can also look specifically at readings at certain times of day, or average readings within various time scales, for example over the last 7 days.

What your results mean

Q What can I do if I regularly get high readings?

You can identify the cause by looking at the times when your readings are high and considering what you were doing in the hours leading up to this. Once you've done this assessment, the next step is taking some action to remedy the situation. You might decide, for example, to decrease the amount of food you eat or increase the amount of physical activity you do.

Q I hurt my back while gardening and have needed to rest. My test results have all been over 15 millimoles per litre since. What should I do?

Your blood glucose level is likely to be high because you are inactive, so temporarily increasing the dose of your tablets or insulin (if you are using medication) will bring it down again. When you are better and become active again, your blood glucose level is likely to fall, so you may need to decrease the dose of your medication at this point. You can also increase your tablets or insulin dose like this when you are ill or when you gain weight – when you recover or lose weight you can adjust your dose down again.

Q My blood glucose keeps swinging between high and low readings – what should I do?

This sometimes happens when you have a "hypo" and treat it with glucose or a sugary snack. Because your liver also releases glucose to compensate for the hypo, you end up with a high level of glucose in your blood. Reducing your medication, or altering your activity levels or eating patterns, can help you to avoid hypos. Other causes of a swinging blood glucose level are an irregular daily routine or food intake, or variations in the timing or dose of your medication. Thinking about these possibilities will help you to identify the cause.

SOME REASONS FOR HIGHS AND LOWS

The occasional high or low blood glucose reading doesn't mean your diabetes is out of control (although treating a low blood glucose as soon as possible will prevent it dropping lower). However, if you notice a pattern to your highs and lows, finding out why they are happening can help you take corrective action. The following is a list of possible reasons.

HIGH READINGS	LOW READINGS
Having more food than usual or a different type of food. (A specific food may be the cause if it is associated with high readings on several different occasions).	Having less food than usual, or taking your insulin or tablets and then being unable to eat when you had planned.
Illness and stress can cause a high blood glucose reading because of the effect of the hormones released at these times.	Stress can make your blood glucose level fall if you respond to it by using up more energy or eating less than usual.
Forgetting to take your tablets or your insulin or taking a dose that is too low for you.	Taking an extra dose of tablets, injecting more insulin than you need, or being on too high a dose of tablets or insulin.
Putting on weight.	Losing weight.
Having a hypo earlier in the day, which you treated with glucose.	Drinking a lot of alcohol without eating carbohydrate-containing food at the same time or reducing your medication.
Being less physically active than usual.	Being more physically active than usual.

Q How often does my blood glucose need to be high before I should worry about it?

A one-off or occasional high reading with an obvious cause will not cause long-term damage to your nerves or blood vessels, but if you have high readings for more than a day or two, then it's worth trying to identify the cause and taking remedial action.

Q What can I do if I get a lot of low readings?

Your monitoring diary will help you to identify what you were doing – in terms of activity, eating, drinking, or taking medication – before your low readings. Once you have found out the reason for the low readings you can decide what action to take to prevent them recurring. If you are unsure what steps you should take, talking to your health professional might help you work out what to do.

Q Can low readings do any harm?

Repeated low readings can mean you are less safe while driving or can reduce your awareness of when you are starting to have a hypo (see pp172–175). This lack of awareness is dangerous because if you are not able to react to the early warning signs of your hypo you will be less able to treat yourself. Taking action quickly in response to low readings, such as having a glucose drink, will help to keep or restore your warning symptoms. Avoiding hypos altogether for a few weeks can also help to restore your symptoms.

Q Is it okay to round my test results up or down to make whole numbers in my diary?

Yes. The range of your results is more important than the exact tenth of a millimole that the decimal point indicates. If you have a reading of 7.4 you can round down to 7, while if you have a reading of 7.5 or more then you could round up to the next whole number, in this example 8.

The HbA1c test

What is an HbA1c test?

The HbA1c test (each letter is pronounced separately) provides information about your blood glucose level. It measures the amount of glucose attached to the haemoglobin (oxygen-carrying molecule) in your blood and gives an average picture of your blood glucose level over the previous 6–8 weeks. The test involves having a blood sample taken from your arm or finger. The sample is then analysed in a laboratory or in the clinic. The HbA1c test is not affected by what you have eaten or drunk in the last few days.

How often do I need an HbA1c test?

Your HbA1c test is taken at least once a year. You might need more frequent tests if, for example, your medication has changed or to assess the effect of any lifestyle changes you have made. Unless you are pregnant, you are unlikely to have an HbA1c test more frequently than every 2 months because it takes this amount of time for the results to change significantly.

What do my HbA1c test results mean?

HbA1c results are given as a percentage – the closer they are to 6.5 per cent (or below), the nearer you are to everyday blood glucose results between 4 and 7 millimoles per litre. If your HbA1c result is above 6.5 per cent, discussing your diabetes management with your health professional can help you decide what needs to change. Every 1 per cent rise in your HbA1c result increases the risk of long-term complications by 30 per cent – so taking steps to keep your HbA1c level at or below 6.5 per cent is of great long-term benefit.

Q If I have a result of 6.5 per cent or lower, will this prevent the long-term complications of diabetes?

Your HbA1c is only one factor that influences your risk, but it is an important one. It is impossible to guarantee that you will never develop the long-term complications of diabetes, such as eye and kidney problems, but the more time your HbA1c is below 6.5 per cent the higher your chance of staying healthy, and the risk of your developing these problems is greatly reduced.

Q I'm hoping to get pregnant. Do I need an HbA1c test beforehand?

Yes, your health professional will check your HbA1c if you are planning a baby. High readings can affect your baby's development, so working to achieve a reading below 6.5 per cent before you conceive is very important.

Q My home blood glucose tests are usually in the range 4–7 millimoles per litre. Will my HbA1c level be around 6.5 per cent?

Your HbA1c test is a measure of your blood glucose levels at all times of the day, so if you don't do home tests very often, you may be falsely reassured by results that are in the 4–7 millimoles per litre range. However, if you test at least once or twice a day and all your results are in the recommended range, your HbA1c level will be close to or below 6.5 per cent.

Q Can I buy a home HbA1c testing kit?

You can buy a home HbA1c testing kit at some pharmacies. It might be useful to discuss with your health professional whether home HbA1c testing would benefit you before you buy a kit.

Q My tests are all under 10 millimoles per litre, but my HbA1c is 12 per cent. Why is this?

Although your results are below 10 millimoles per litre at the times you do them, they may be higher at other times. This will affect your HbA1c result. Varying the times you test, for example, after meals as well as before, and aiming for results between 4–7 millimoles per litre, helps to influence your HbA1c result.

Understanding your blood pressure

My doctor tested me for Type 2 diabetes because I am having treatment for high blood pressure. Why is that?

Type 2 diabetes and high blood pressure are both linked to insulin resistance, so if you have one of these conditions it is common to have the other, too. Keeping both your blood pressure and your blood glucose level under control means that your chances of developing long-term complications, especially heart disease, are greatly reduced.

What is high blood pressure?

If your larger blood vessels become more rigid and your smaller blood vessels start to constrict, your blood has to flow through a narrower space than before. The result is greater pressure on your blood vessel walls, which is known as high blood pressure or, medically, as hypertension. Having high blood pressure is common when you have Type 2 diabetes.

I have high blood pressure but I don't feel ill. Why does it need to be treated?

Having high blood pressure makes you much more prone to cardiovascular disease (CVD) – a serious condition that develops over many years as your blood vessels gradually become narrower and less flexible. You may have high blood pressure without knowing it and, if it remains untreated, you may develop angina (severe chest pain) or have a heart attack or a stroke. Taking your blood pressure treatment as prescribed and having regular check-ups can help prevent these serious conditions.

Myth "You know if you have high blood pressure because it gives you headaches"

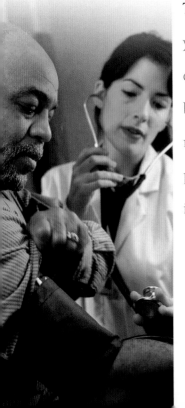

Truth High blood pressure does not always give you symptoms, and it is often found by chance during routine health checks. Having your blood pressure checked at your annual diabetes reviews, and more frequently if your health professional suggests it, will be a more reliable indicator of whether your blood pressure is high.

What should my blood pressure be?

If you have Type 2 diabetes your blood pressure should be below 140/80 millimetres of mercury (mmHg). In some situations, for example if you have already developed kidney damage (nephropathy), you may need to keep your blood pressure lower, for example, 135/75 millimetres of mercury (mmHg) to prevent further damage. Discussing your ideal blood pressure level, and ways to achieve it, with your health professional will give you the level that is right for you.

Why are there two figures in my blood pressure measurement?

The top figure refers to the level of pressure in your blood vessels as your heart contracts and pumps blood around your body. This is known as the systolic blood pressure. The second figure is the lowest pressure as your heart relaxes between beats. This is known as the diastolic blood pressure.

What can I do to lower my blood pressure?

Stopping smoking and losing weight if you need to, eating more fresh fruit and vegetables and less salt (for example, less processed or ready meals) will help to reduce your blood pressure. Staying active or becoming more active (see pp78–97) will also lower your blood pressure. Taking any blood pressure tablets that you have been prescribed, even if they do not affect the way you feel, will help keep your blood pressure in the recommended range.

How low can my blood pressure go?

It would be unusual for your blood pressure to be under 100/60 mmHg if you are otherwise healthy. For every 10 mmHg drop in your systolic blood pressure (the first figure) towards this level, you benefit by reducing your risk of heart attack or stroke.

Monitoring blood pressure

Q How often should I have my blood pressure checked?

Your blood pressure will be checked at least once a year at your annual review (see pp120–121). If you have high blood pressure, you will probably have frequent checks, for example, every 1–4 weeks. Once stable, your blood pressure will be checked every 3–6 months.

Q How will my blood pressure be measured?

Your health professional will wrap a cuff around your upper arm and inflate it either manually or with an electronic device, until it is tight enough to prevent blood flowing to your lower arm. The cuff is then slowly deflated and your blood pressure is measured by the electronic device or by your health professional listening to the blood flow in your arm with a stethoscope. The two figures in your blood pressure measurement refer, firstly, to the pressure in your blood vessel as your heart contracts (systolic blood pressure) and, secondly, to when your heart is relaxed (diastolic blood pressure).

Q I am always anxious when I visit my clinic – will that raise my blood pressure?

Your blood pressure goes up and down depending on the time of the day and your stress levels. If you feel anxious about seeing your health professional, your blood pressure rises. This is why your blood pressure may be checked two or three times – or for 24 hours – before you are diagnosed with high blood pressure.

Q Can I measure my blood pressure at home?

Yes, but talking to your health professional before buying your own monitor may give you useful information, or you may be able to borrow a monitor from them if you need one for a short time.

If I want to monitor my own blood pressure, how often should I do it?

How often you check your blood pressure depends on what you want to know. For example, if you want to find out how a stressful situation affects your blood pressure, take "before and after" readings. If you simply want to know whether your blood pressure is in the recommended range, take readings several times a day for a few days to establish what is normal for you. After this, checking your blood pressure occasionally, for example once or twice a week, will be enough.

How do I use my electronic monitor?

Your monitor will contain specific instructions on how to use it – the exact position of the cuff or your arm varies from monitor to monitor. Once you start the monitor, the cuff will automatically inflate and deflate and then the monitor will give you a reading of your blood pressure. Sitting down for 5–10 minutes before you measure your blood pressure will increase the accuracy of the reading.

What do I do if I get readings that seem to be higher than my recommended range?

Occasional high readings can be due to stress or life events such as a busy day or pressure at work, but if you are regularly having high readings, you may need to have your treatment started, or reviewed and changed. With Type 2 diabetes, you may need three or more different types of tablets to control your blood pressure (see pp160–161). Other factors that can raise your blood pressure are eating a lot of salt and being very inactive. Tackling any of these factors can help to lower your blood pressure – for example, you could regularly do relaxation exercises, you could increase your activity levels, or you could prepare more meals yourself instead of eating processed food.

Your annual review

Q What is an annual review?

Once a year, your health professional will assess with you how well your blood glucose level and blood pressure are controlled and check for any signs of the long-term complications of diabetes. Many of the tests are the same as those that were carried out shortly after your diagnosis. You will also have the opportunity to discuss any problems or concerns at your review.

Q How can I get the most from my annual review?

Writing down any questions or concerns you have and taking them to your review will help you to remember them. During the review, make a note of any changes to your tablets or insulin or other medications you are taking. You may also find it useful to write down what any change in treatment is for, how quickly treatment will work, and what side effects you should look out for, and what action to take should side effects occur.

Q What happens if any of my tests are outside the expected range?

You may need changes to your diabetes treatment or other medications to bring your test results back into the recommended range. If you have signs of long-term complications (with your eyes or feet, for example), you will be referred to a specialist.

Q What should I do if I'm not sure whether I've had all the tests I need?

Your main medical records will have a comprehensive record of your overall health and should contain information about your latest results. If you want to check that you have had all the tests, you can make an appointment with your health professional about 3 weeks after your annual review.

When do I get my test results?

Some of your tests provide information immediately – for example, your blood pressure or your feet being examined. Others, such as blood tests, may take a week or two before your results are available.

What if I need help in between my annual reviews?

Contact your health professional if you have problems such as frequent hypos, a consistently high blood glucose level, foot injuries that are not healing, sudden changes in your vision, problems with medication or equipment, or feeling unable to cope with your diabetes. He or she can give information, arrange tests, and make sure you see any other health professionals you need to.

MEDICAL TESTS AT YOUR ANNUAL REVIEW

Blood pressure check	Identifies how well your blood pressure is controlled.
Eye examination or photograph	Identifies any damage to the retina (the light sensitive part at the backs of your eyes).
Foot check	Assesses whether you have poor circulation and/or reduced sensation in your feet.
Weight and waist and hip measurements	Assesses whether your weight or body shape increases your risk of cardiovascular disease (CVD).
Urine test	Tests for the presence of protein in your urine, which may be a sign of kidney damage.
Blood tests	Several different tests are made on blood samples to assess your overall blood glucose control, your blood fats, and your kidney function.

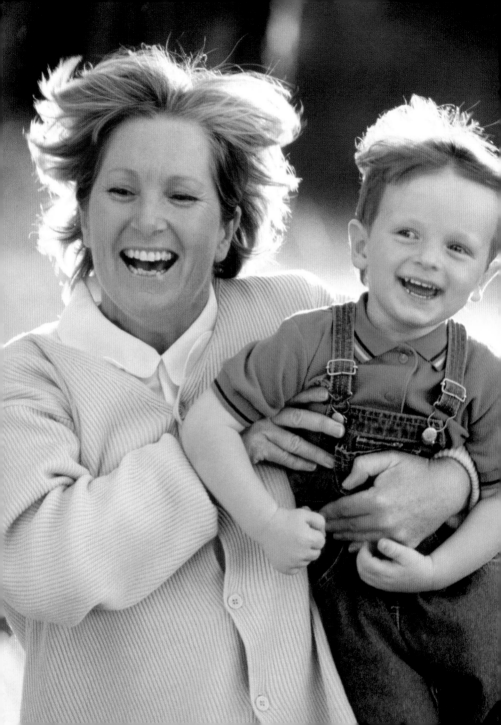

Living with diabetes

Taking good care of your feet, managing stress, and knowing what to do when you are ill are all important aspects of your day-to-day life with diabetes. If you are a woman, pregnancy and the menopause will also affect your diabetes. If you live with, or are close to, someone who has Type 2 diabetes, you will find information on the condition and support helpful in day-to-day life.

Day-to-day life

Q How will having diabetes affect my work?

Hopefully, very little, with some forward planning. You may find it helpful to develop a plan for testing, eating, or adjusting your medication that fits into your working day. If your job is unpredictable or involves a lot of physical activity, you may need to check your blood glucose several times during the day. If your job is sedentary, this may cause your blood glucose level to rise. If appropriate, you may find it helpful to keep supplies of medication and hypo remedies at work.

Q Are there any jobs that I won't be able to do?

Yes, there are a few jobs that are not open to you. They include entering the army, navy, or air force, and flying commercial aircraft. If you take insulin, you cannot hold or continue to hold a large goods vehicle or public service vehicle licence. Otherwise, if you take insulin or insulin-stimulating tablets (meaning you are risk of hypos) and you are responsible for the safety of others, you must tell your employer that you have diabetes.

Q Can I still drive?

If your treatment consists of healthy eating and physical activity, you do not need to inform the Driver and Vehicle Licensing Authority (DVLA) about your diabetes. If you take tablets or insulin, you have to notify the DVLA and your insurance company. If you take insulin, your licence will be restricted to 1, 2, or 3 years, and you will not be able to hold a large goods vehicle or passenger-carrying vehicle licence. If you already have either of these types of licence, and you start insulin treatment, your licence will be revoked.

I sometimes have hypos. How should I deal with a long drive?

Testing your blood glucose before you drive, and about every 2 hours during the journey will tell you if your blood glucose is within the recommended range. Keeping supplies of food, drink, and hypo remedies in the car means you have supplies readily available.

I travel abroad a lot. How will this affect my diabetes?

Long distance and air travel, changes in time zones, temperature, and different food, drinks, or activities when you are abroad will all affect your blood glucose level, even if you do not take any medication for your diabetes. You can help prevent problems by making sure that your travel insurance covers any diabetes-related problems, and packing enough supplies of your equipment and medication (they may not be available in other countries). If you are flying, ask your health professional for a letter explaining to the airline that you need to keep your diabetes equipment in your hand luggage. Detailed planning ahead will help you manage your diabetes safely during your trips.

Can I still go on my regular night out now I have diabetes?

Having diabetes will not stop you from doing anything you enjoyed before. If you drink a lot of alcohol on your night out and you take insulin or insulin–stimulating tablets, you will need to protect yourself from hypos (see pp126–129).

Which organizations can I contact for advice about diabetes?

National organizations such as Diabetes UK have a telephone care line, a website, and they publish a range of leaflets and magazines with up-to-date information about all aspects of diabetes. See p200 for contact details of Diabetes UK and other organizations that may provide you with useful advice and information.

Dealing with hypoglycaemia

Q What is a hypo?

A hypo, or hypoglycaemic attack, is when your blood glucose level falls below 4 millimoles per litre. This happens when you have more insulin working in your body than you need. Your symptoms (see below) should warn you that your blood glucose level is low, although if your body is accustomed to blood glucose levels below 4 millimoles per litre, your symptoms may be reduced or absent.

Q What would I feel like if I had a hypo?

When your blood glucose level is between 3–4 millimoles per litre, you may get symptoms such as palpitations, sweating, trembling, feeling anxious, turning pale, and hunger. If your blood glucose level falls below 3 millimoles per litre, your symptoms alter as your brain starts to be deprived of glucose and no longer functions well. You might feel disorientated, find it difficult to concentrate, have blurred vision or a headache. You may also be uncooperative or aggressive.

Q How likely am I to have a hypo?

You are at risk of hypos only if you take insulin or insulin-stimulating tablets, such as sulphonylureas. (If you manage your diabetes with other types of tablets, or with activity and healthy eating, you will not have hypos.) Several factors can increase the risk of a hypo, for example, being more active than usual or having an imbalance of your tablets or insulin and carbohydrate-containing food. Weight loss also makes hypos more likely – if you lose weight you will probably need a lower dose of tablets or insulin.

How can I prevent myself having a hypo?

Identifying situations where you are at risk of hypos, for example, eating less, drinking alcohol, or being in a hot climate/environment, such as a hot bath or sauna, will help you plan ahead. In these situations, carrying extra snacks or reducing your insulin/tablet dose in advance means you are prepared if your blood glucose drops. If it helps, ask friends, family, or colleagues to remind you to test your blood glucose or to eat snacks. If you suspect that your blood glucose level is falling at any time, a blood test will give you the information you need to take action.

My blood glucose sometimes drops below 4 but I feel fine. Do I need to do anything?

Yes, any blood glucose level below 4 millimoles per litre is defined as a hypo, regardless of how you are feeling. If you don't get symptoms – or you used to, but don't any more – keeping your blood glucose out of the hypo range for a few weeks can help to restore your symptoms. If you have hypo symptoms and a test result of 4 millimoles per litre, don't wait for your blood glucose to drop below 4 – treat yourself for hypoglycaemia immediately.

How should I treat a hypo?

The initial treatment for a hypo is to eat or drink something that is high in fast-acting carbohydrate. The options include: three or more glucose tablets (available from pharmacies); a high-energy sugar drink, ordinary cola, or lemonade; 2–4 teaspoons of sugar dissolved in water; or 10–20g of glucose or dextrose gel (available from pharmacies). Following this by eating a slower-acting carbohydrate food will help to keep your blood glucose level up. Options include a sandwich, a piece of toast, a piece of fruit, two biscuits, or a bowl of cereal.

Q Will I become unconscious or pass out if I have a hypo?

If you don't treat or receive treatment for your hypo and your blood glucose level continues to fall, you may lose consciousness, although this is rare. It usually takes up to 2 hours or more after your early warning symptoms start – but it may happen within 10–15 minutes of the later symptoms. If you lose consciousness and you don't receive help, your body will usually gradually recover by itself, and you regain consciousness naturally within an hour or two.

TREATING A HYPO

A family member or friend who takes insulin or insulin-stimulating tablets may have a hypo from time to time. If the person is confused and unable to treat himself, you may need to help. Follow these two steps as long as the person is conscious. If the person loses consciousness, you may need to give a glucagon injection (see right).

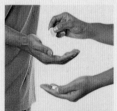

① If the person has early symptoms of a hypo, such as sweating, trembling, or palpitations, ask him to do a blood glucose test. If he has later symptoms of a hypo, such as confusion, aggression, or blurred vision, ask him to eat three or more glucose tablets or drink a sugary drink immediately.

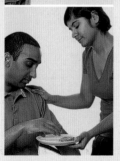

② If the person starts to feel better quickly, give a carbohydrate snack to keep his blood glucose level up after the glucose has been absorbed. This could be a couple of biscuits, a sandwich, or a bowl of cereal. Too much carbohydrate food can cause a high blood glucose level later. Stay with the person until he or she feels better. Don't give any food or drink to someone you suspect is losing consciousness in case he or she is unable to swallow.

One of my friends has a glucagon injection kit at home. Should I have one?

Glucagon is sometimes used to treat serious hypos – it works by converting glycogen in your liver to glucose. If you have good early warning symptoms of hypos, you do not need a glucagon kit, as you will have plenty of time to take glucose followed by a carbohydrate snack. If you don't get the early symptoms of a hypo, or you tend to become disorientated or lose consciousness very quickly, it might be a good idea to get a glucagon kit so that a colleague, friend, or family member can inject you with glucagon if necessary. If you are unsure about whether you need a glucagon kit, consulting your health professional will help you to decide.

What will happen to me if I have a hypo in the middle of the night when I am asleep?

You may wake up, but even if you carry on sleeping, your body will eventually correct your blood glucose level by converting glycogen in your liver into glucose and releasing it into your bloodstream. Excess insulin also wears off naturally in time. Hypos can, rarely, be life-threatening if you have been drinking large amounts of alcohol on an empty stomach, because alcohol impairs this corrective mechanism. This is why it is essential to balance your alcohol intake with food or to take a lower dose of insulin or insulin-stimulating tablets if you know that you are going to be drinking.

Sometimes after a hypo my blood glucose goes really high. Does this mean I've eaten too much?

Not necessarily. Your liver responds to a hypo by releasing extra glucose into your bloodstream, which can make your blood glucose rise too high after you have had a hypo. Eating 20–30g of a carbohydrate food should be sufficient to treat your hypo – eating a greater amount than this can contribute to your high blood glucose reading.

Dealing with hyperglycaemia

Q What is hyperglycaemia?

Hyperglycaemia is when your blood glucose level rises above 7 millimoles per litre. You probably had hyperglycaemia when you were first diagnosed with diabetes. You may also have it if your treatment – healthy eating, physical activity, taking tablets, and/or insulin – is not working effectively enough.

Q What will I feel like if I get hyperglycaemia?

You may have symptoms such as a dry mouth, excessive thirst, passing large amounts of urine frequently, fatigue, and blurred vision. However, these symptoms usually only appear when your blood glucose level is 10 millimoles or more. If you want to know if your blood glucose is rising above 7 millimoles per litre, the only way to tell is by doing blood glucose tests.

Q I still feel well even though my blood glucose is between 10 and 15 millimoles per litre. Is that OK?

No, you still need to take action to lower your blood glucose level. A regularly raised blood glucose level will increase your risk of developing long-term complications (see pp180–199). Also, if your body becomes accustomed to a higher-than-normal blood glucose level, you may not get symptoms until your blood glucose level reaches 15 millimoles per litre or more. So, even if you are feeling well, testing your blood glucose level regularly rather than waiting for symptoms is the only way to reliably detect hyperglycaemia.

If my blood glucose is well controlled does that mean I will never have hyperglycaemia?

No. There will be times when you have readings of more than 7 millimoles per litre, for example, after a celebratory meal, if you are less active than usual, or during an illness or infection. Occasional high readings will not do you any harm, but regular high readings should prompt you to take action.

What should I do if I keep getting a high blood glucose level?

Try to identify what is causing your hyperglycaemia. Work out if it is related to your food intake or reduced physical activity on a particular day, and take appropriate action by, for example, eating less or being more active. If there are no obvious causes of your raised blood glucose level, you may need to start taking tablets (if you don't already take them), increase the dose of your tablets, or start injecting insulin. Your health professional can help decide what action to take.

How can I prevent hyperglycaemia?

Preventive measures include taking your tablets or insulin every day, avoiding foods that make your blood glucose rise too high, or compensating for eating these foods by adjusting your medication or being more active. If you are aware of the effect of stress and other hormonal changes on your blood glucose, this can help you predict when you will need to adjust your treatment. To prevent hyperglycaemia during illness, don't stop taking your insulin (especially if you are vomiting) or tablets . If your tablets or insulin don't keep your blood glucose level in the recommended range during an illness, you may need an increased dose. See pp142–145 for more information on illness. Regular blood glucose testing can also warn you of hyperglycaemia.

Looking after your heart

Q What can I do to keep my heart and circulation healthy?

The most important things you can do are to stay or become active, eat healthily (see pp46–47 and pp78–79), and to stop smoking and lose weight if you need to. Also, taking any prescribed treatment will help to keep your blood glucose, blood pressure, and blood fat levels within healthy limits.

Q I've had so much advice about what to eat – what are the most important things to remember?

Eating healthy types of fats, for example, monounsaturated fat rather than saturated fat, and limiting your overall fat intake will help to protect your heart. High-calorie foods can cause weight gain, which in turn will increase your risk of heart disease, so trying to keep your calorie intake within the recommended limits will help (see pp72–74). If you have high blood pressure, keeping the amount of salt you eat low (see p52) is useful. Eating foods that are rich in antioxidants, such as fruit, vegetables, wholegrains and pulses, and eating oily fish twice a week, can help protect against heart disease (see pp46–47).

Q What sort of exercise will help reduce my risk of heart disease?

Any aerobic activities – those that increase your heart rate and make you feel warm and slightly out of breath – such as walking, swimming, or digging the garden, are all good for your heart. If you haven't been active for a long time, see pp88–91 for ideas on how to get started. If you already have a heart problem, physical activity is likely to improve your health, but your health professional can help you decide which activities will most benefit you.

What help can I get to stop smoking?

Your health professional can help you to find local stopping smoking clinics. You may be asked to attend on a regular basis to talk about how you are coping, or you may be offered information about using nicotine replacement therapy (such as patches or chewing gum) to help deal with your cravings. You can also buy self-help books that you might find useful.

My doctor has prescribed eight different tablets. Do I really need to take all of them?

Type 2 diabetes is a complex disease and you probably have a number of conditions: a high blood glucose level, high blood pressure, and a high level of blood fats, often accompanied by being overweight. Each one of these increases your chance of developing heart disease, so you may have been prescribed tablets for each of these. You may need two or more types of tablet just to control your blood glucose level and possibly insulin as well; you may need three or more different types of tablets to treat your blood pressure (see pp160–161); and you may need more tablets to lower your blood fat levels. In addition to these, you may be prescribed aspirin to protect your heart, and tablets to reduce your appetite.

I've already had a heart attack. Is there any point trying to keep healthy?

Your heart attack shows that heart disease has already done some damage, but taking steps towards better health will prevent this getting worse and improve the health of your heart. Taking action now, such as becoming more active and giving up smoking if you smoke, will greatly reduce your chances of having another heart attack or a stroke. Your heart is able to recover, and each step you take towards healthier living will help.

Myth "I will know if my nerves are damaged because my feet will be more painful"

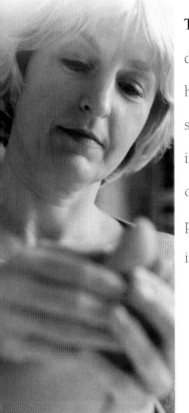

Truth When the nerves to your feet become damaged, this alters your ability to feel what's happening to them. You might get different sensations from normal, such as tingling, but in general you will have less feeling, so burning or damaging your feet won't cause you much pain. The amount of pain you have is not a good indication of whether you have nerve damage.

Looking after your feet

Why do I need to look after my feet?

Over time, diabetes can reduce the efficiency of your blood circulation and nervous system, which can affect many areas of your body, including your feet. This makes you more prone to foot ulcers and other injuries. These can become infected. You can prevent serious problems by looking after your feet carefully.

If there is something wrong with my feet, will they be painful?

Not necessarily – if the nerves supplying your feet have been damaged, you may have reduced sensation. You may experience tingling feelings in your feet, but not be aware of an injury or other problem until it is quite advanced. Checking your feet all over every day is the only sure way to tell if something is wrong. You may need to enlist someone else's help if you can't do this yourself, for example, if your eyesight is poor or you have problems bending to reach your feet.

How should I look after my feet?

The box on p137 shows you how to check, wash, dry, and moisturize your feet on a day-to-day basis. In addition to this, taking precautions such as not walking barefoot, particularly when you are outside or in unfamiliar surroundings, will help prevent you damaging your feet.

Can I cut my toenails myself?

Yes, see the box on p137 for advice on nail cutting. However, if you have reduced feeling or circulation in your feet, check with your health professional whether you can cut your nails safely. If you can't bend to cut your nails, or they are too thick, you may need help.

Q What sort of footwear do I need?

Try to avoid wearing tight or restrictive socks or tights. It's also a good idea to avoid pointed toes and high heels for everyday wear – your footwear should not rub or cramp any areas of your feet. Check inside your footwear to make sure there are no sharp objects sticking through the soles.

Q What should I do if I have a blister?

Try to leave blisters alone. Don't pop them, and avoid putting pressure on them. If a blister bursts, cover it with a piece of gauze and tape and keep checking it to make sure it heals. Consult your health professional if a blister is not healing properly.

Q Do I need to take any special precautions when I go rambling?

It's a good idea to invest in a pair of good quality shoes or boots that support the length and width of your feet. Leather is an ideal material since it moulds to the shape of your feet. Check your feet carefully before you go rambling and when you come back. It's useful to carry a basic first aid kit with you in case you get a blister.

Q When should I seek professional help for foot injuries?

All but the most minor foot problems should be treated by a health professional. You can treat athlete's foot by yourself at home using an antifungal cream or powder, but you should seek help for all of the following: corns, ingrowing toenails, hard or cracked skin, sore areas that don't seem to be healing, bruising or discoloration, and any loss of feeling in any part of your foot.

Q Can I put a hot water bottle on my feet?

It's not advisable to put your feet against any direct source of heat, whether it's a hot water bottle or a radiator, because of the risk of burns. If your feet get cold in bed, wear a pair of loose-fitting socks.

DAY-TO-DAY FOOT CARE

A good foot-care routine will help you to keep your feet healthy. Carrying out this procedure every day, allowing plenty of time to thoroughly check your feet for injuries and problems, will help you to spot potential problems early on.

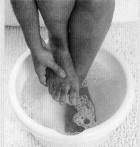

① Wash your feet daily in warm water, using a mild soap. Avoid soaking your feet for more than 10 minutes, however, because this can dry out the skin.

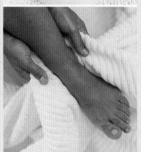

② Dry your feet carefully, especially in between your toes. Now check for tender areas, bruising, and cuts or hard or cracked skin on the top and on the soles of your feet. Trim your toenails when you need to. Cut them to the shape of and level with the end of your toe. Don't cut them too short and don't stick sharp instruments down the side of a nail.

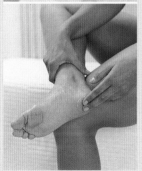

③ Apply an unperfumed moisturizing cream to your feet, paying attention to the skin between your toes and any hard skin on your soles.

Stress and diabetes

Q I sometimes feel irritable – is this the same thing as stress?

Short-term irritability may be normal for you, but if you're irritable most of the time, you are probably suffering from stress. Being constantly annoyed or irritated, feeling pressured, and finding it difficult to make day-to-day decisions about your life and your diabetes are all signs of stress. Try to find out what is causing your stress in order to find ways to deal with it – see the action plan on p141.

Q What signs of stress should I look out for?

Stress affects people in different ways. You may have physical symptoms such as tension headaches, migraines, digestive problems, or insomnia. Your appetite may increase or decrease, and you may have cravings for caffeine, alcohol, or sugary snacks.

Q Can stress cause diabetes?

The hormones you produce when you are stressed or unwell, or after a shock, can make your insulin less effective and cause your blood glucose to rise. If your pancreas has already been struggling to produce enough insulin, stress may be the factor that tips the balance and raises your blood glucose, leading to your diabetes being diagnosed. But stress only exposes underlying diabetes – it doesn't cause it.

Q How will stress affect my diabetes?

Stress hormones tend to cause your blood glucose level to rise (see previous question). If stress is regularly causing high blood glucose – even if this is short-term – you may need an increase in your medication. If you are unsure of what to do, ask your health professional.

How can I beat stress?

Relaxation can provide a longer-term solution to stress than more instant solutions, such as smoking, drinking coffee or alcohol, or eating comfort foods. If it's difficult to take any time out to reduce your stress, talk to someone close to you and ask for their help and support. The four-step action plan on p141 can help you to find ways of coping.

Can physical activity reduce stress?

Yes, being active raises your levels of endorphins and serotonin, two brain chemicals that influence your mood and sense of wellbeing. If you can fit physical activity into your life on a regular basis, you will feel better all round. Being active helps your body to work more efficiently and raises your self-esteem. See pp78–97 for information on becoming and staying active.

How can relaxation help me be less stressed?

Unlike quick-fixes, such as alcohol, coffee, cigarettes, or sugary comfort food, relaxation is a solution to stress that will help you to cope better in the long-term. Taking time to relax can help you to put things into perspective. Deep breathing, stretching, a walk in the fresh air, or listening to your favourite music can all help to reduce stress.

When I'm stressed I find it difficult to look after my diabetes. What can I do?

Stress can reduce your ability to cope with daily tasks, including looking after your diabetes. You may also feel you want to over-eat or eat less healthily when you are stressed. Try to set yourself small realistic goals during these times, for example, eating two or three portions of fruit and vegetables a day or limiting how many biscuits you eat. Feeling that you can still meet one or two small goals will help you to stay motivated.

How to manage stress

Diabetes is a lifelong condition and at times it's normal to feel frustrated or fed up about the effort it takes to look after yourself. Being aware of stress, and taking action quickly, can prevent things getting on top of you. Dealing with stress can also help your blood glucose control. When you are under stress, your body produces hormones that make your insulin even less effective – this is why it's important to closely monitor your blood glucose level at times of stress. Physical activity is a useful way of relieving stress – and it lowers your blood glucose, too.

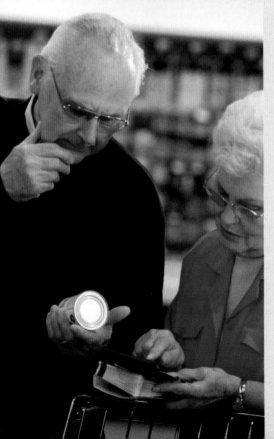

SOURCES OF DIABETES-RELATED STRESS

Working hard to control your diabetes but still getting high blood glucose readings.

Feeling guilty because you haven't found time to monitor your blood glucose level.

Finding it hard to remember to take your medication at the right times.

Being in situations where you don't have access to the sort of food you need.

Conflict between the way you manage your diabetes and the way other people – friends and family, for example – tell you you should be managing your diabetes.

Guilt about being inactive or overweight.

Feeling fed up with your day-to-day diabetes routine.

LEARNING TO RELAX

Yoga is a great way to calm your mind, and you don't have to spend lots of time learning complicated poses. Some simple stretching movements combined with breathing exercises can quickly make you feel calmer.

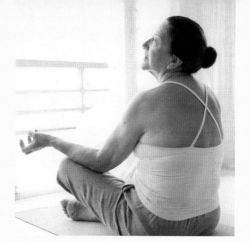

ACTION PLAN TO BEAT DIABETES-RELATED STRESS

If you feel the stress of looking after your diabetes is getting on top of you, this four-step action plan can help. Checking your progress will help you see if you are achieving your goals. You might want to reward yourself if you are doing well, or revise your plan if you are still struggling.

① What situations are causing stress in your life?

Identify the times when you find it difficult to look after your diabetes, and which tasks present the biggest challenge. Be as specific as possible about what is stressful.

② What are your feelings?

Consider how you feel about situations that cause you stress and write your feelings down. Acknowledging that you feel anxious, resentful, or angry about some aspects of your diabetes care is often the first step to tackling this.

③ What are your options?

Identify how you would like to care for your diabetes then ask yourself what steps you could take to be in this position. For example, if you are worried about not doing enough blood glucose tests, what changes in your life would enable you to test more frequently?

④ What are you going to do?

Work out what exactly you are going to do on a week-to-week basis with targets and a time scale. Keeping your action plan to hand will remind you of these.

When you are ill

Q Am I more prone to infections because I have diabetes?

Simply having diabetes does not make you more prone to common illnesses than anyone else. But if your blood glucose level is consistently high – for example, more than 10 millimoles per litre – this increases your vulnerability to infection because it's an ideal environment for bacteria and viruses to thrive.

Q How does an infection, such as a cold or flu, affect my blood glucose level?

An infection is likely to raise your blood glucose level. This is because part of your body's natural reaction to illness is to produce more glucose. You also produce stress hormones such as adrenaline and cortisol which make your natural or injected insulin less efficient at controlling your blood glucose level. So, even if you are not eating any food, your blood glucose level is likely to be raised.

Q What should I do about my diabetes if I become ill?

Testing your blood glucose level at least every four hours will tell you whether it is above 10 millimoles per litre – if it is, you will need to adjust your medication. If you feel too ill to do blood tests or you are unsure what to do, consult your health professional sooner rather than later.

Q What should I do about eating and drinking when I am ill?

Try not to stop eating and drinking – you need food and liquid to help you fight illness, prevent dehydration, and keep your temperature down. Drink at least 2 litres of sugar-free fluids every day to prevent dehydration. If you are being uncontrollably sick, contact your health professional urgently.

If I can't eat when I'm ill, should I still take my tablets and insulin?

Yes, your body produces glucose even if you are not eating, and it may produce more glucose than usual when you are ill. Continuing to take your tablets or insulin is essential to keep your blood glucose level down, and you may even need to temporarily increase your dose. You can reduce the dose when you recover. If you have a longer-term illness, taking your medication to keep your blood glucose within the recommended range will help to prevent the long-term complications of diabetes.

I usually take cough medicine and flu remedies when I'm ill. Can I still do this?

Drugs and remedies that you buy over the counter are safe to use when you have diabetes. Even drugs that contain sugar, such as cough syrup, will not have a significant effect on your blood glucose level because the dose that you will need to take is fairly small. If you prefer, you can ask your pharmacist to recommend a low-sugar product.

What effect would a stomach upset have on my blood glucose?

Bouts of sickness and diarrhoea may be short-lived, but they can have a serious effect on your diabetes within the space of a few hours. The main danger is that your blood glucose level can rise very high, causing severe dehydration. Doing regular blood glucose tests – or asking someone to do this for you if you are not well enough – will give you information about your diabetes control and when to contact your health professional.

Is it true that severe dehydration can lead to a coma?

Severe dehydration can lead to a condition known as non-ketotic hyperosmolar state (HONK), which may result in a coma. This is why, if you can't take your tablets or keep food or fluids down, you should contact your health professional or hospital as soon as possible.

Drugs for long-term illness

Q I take tablets for high blood pressure. Will these affect my diabetes control?

Certain tablets you may be prescribed for high blood pressure, including thiazide diuretics such as bendroflumethiazide, and beta blockers such as propranolol, can affect your blood glucose level. You might need two or three different types of tablets in combination to treat your high blood pressure effectively. Even if your blood pressure tablets affect your blood glucose, you still need to take them, because reducing your blood pressure is just as important as lowering your blood glucose.

Q Is it true that steroids can affect my blood glucose?

Yes, steroid tablets or injections increase your blood glucose level because they make it harder for your insulin to work effectively. Even if you are only taking steroids for a short time, you may need to increase the dose of your tablets or insulin to compensate. Consult your health professional if you are unsure. Steroids may be prescribed to reduce inflammation if you have Crohn's disease, ulcerative colitis, or rheumatoid arthritis. They are also used to treat chronic lung conditions, such as asthma.

Q My blood pressure tablets affect my blood glucose level but my doctor says they are the ones I need. What can I do?

Controlling your blood pressure is as important as controlling your blood glucose level in terms of preventing the long-term complications of diabetes. If your blood pressure tablets are effective, you may need to work out with your health professional what food or activity changes you can make to control your blood glucose level, or what changes in medication you need.

Going into hospital

I am having an operation unrelated to diabetes. Should I keep up my normal diabetes routine?

If you are asked not to eat or drink anything before your operation, you may need to reduce your dose of tablets or insulin before you go into hospital – consult your health professional about this. Once you are in hospital, the staff will probably take over your diabetes care around the time of your operation. If you have to remain in hospital, you may be able to do your own blood glucose tests and manage your own medication.

What do a glucose drip and an insulin infusion do?

This treatment closely controls your blood glucose level when you are not able to eat properly, for example, when you are having an operation. An insulin infusion and a glucose drip are inserted into your vein – the rate at which insulin enters your bloodstream is adjusted according to your blood glucose level, which is measured every hour. As soon as you are eating properly again, the glucose drip and insulin infusions are replaced with your usual tablets or insulin.

When I'm discharged from hospital should I go back to my old diabetes routine?

During your hospital stay, changes may have been made to your diabetes medication because of the effect of your illness or operation. Before you leave hospital, ask your health professional if your medication has changed or what the effects of the change may be. If you have been far less active in hospital than normal and you take insulin-stimulating tablets or insulin, you might be at risk of a hypo if you continue to take the same dose of medication when you resume your normal life at home.

Women's health

Q Can my hormones affect my blood glucose level?

Yes, during your menstrual cycle, levels of oestrogen and progesterone in your body rise and fall, and this can cause your blood glucose level to also rise and fall. This is because your body's production of insulin may not match the varying hormone levels.

Q My blood glucose level changes just before my period. How should I deal with this?

If your blood glucose level rises before your period, doing some extra physical activity, avoiding eating extra carbohydrates, or increasing the dose of your medication for the few days before your period can all help. If your blood glucose level falls and you have more hypos before your period, it may be useful to eat more carbohydrate foods, or to reduce the dose of your medication, and to carry extra hypo remedies.

Q Can I take the contraceptive pill when I have Type 2 diabetes?

Yes, all contraceptive pills are safe to take when you have diabetes. Sometimes the pill can cause a slight rise in your blood glucose level – but you can adapt your diabetes management to deal with this.

Q I'm menopausal and my blood glucose levels are all over the place. Why is this and what can I do?

During the menopause, your hormone levels are unpredictable and this can affect your blood glucose level. Sometimes changes in your blood glucose level let you know that your hormone levels have changed, and sometimes it works the other way round. Monitoring your blood glucose frequently and recording the results – together with how you are feeling – can give you the information you need to adjust your medication. Talking to your health professional may also be helpful.

Can I take hormone replacement therapy (HRT) if I have diabetes?

Diabetes itself will not stop you from taking HRT for a short time to relieve your menopause symptoms. Taking HRT in the long term is not recommended because it may increase your risk of heart disease. If you have had certain forms of cancer, HRT may not be suitable.

Why do I keep getting cystitis and thrush?

Cystitis (an inflammation of your bladder) and thrush (an overgrowth of fungus in your vagina) can both occur if your blood glucose level is frequently higher than recommended. A raised blood glucose level allows bacteria and fungi to thrive. You can have treatment with antibiotics or antifungal tablets or creams. If you have autonomic neuropathy (see p199) that affects your bladder you may also be more prone to cystitis.

Can I still get pregnant now I've got Type 2 diabetes?

Yes, diabetes does not affect your fertility, but you will need to plan your pregnancy, ideally with your health professional. Changing or stopping your usual medication, and taking insulin as well as checking your kidneys and eyes, is recommended. You will also be advised to take folic acid daily and to attend a diabetes antenatal clinic. If you become pregnant by accident, contact your health professional as soon as you know.

Can I still take my diabetes tablets when I'm pregnant?

You may be able to keep taking metformin (see p158) for a time after you find you are pregnant if your pregnancy is unplanned, but other tablets for Type 2 diabetes are not recommended when you are pregnant (or breastfeeding). Your blood glucose level will rise during pregnancy, and when you need medication to control this, your health professional is likely to recommend insulin injections.

Myth "I am less likely to get pregnant because I have Type 2 diabetes"

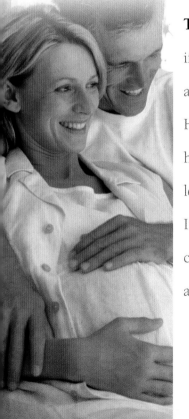

Truth Type 2 diabetes doesn't affect fertility so if you have not yet had your menopause, you are just as likely to become pregnant as before. However, there are risks to yours and your baby's health if you conceive when your blood glucose level is regularly outside the recommended range. If you wish to become pregnant, planning and controlling your blood glucose, blood pressure and cholesterol levels reduce these risks.

How should I care for my diabetes while I'm pregnant?

Aiming for your pre-meal blood glucose level to be between 4–6 millimoles per litre and your post-meal (2 hours after eating) blood glucose level to be 4–7 millimoles per litre, and an HbA1c test result of 6.5 per cent or below, is recommended. As your pregnancy progresses, you will need to take an increased amount of insulin and you will attend regular appointments with your health professional.

Will I need special tests during my pregnancy?

Yes, you will be offered an HbA1c test every 1–2 months, your blood pressure will be taken on every visit to your health professional, and your eyes will be checked at least every three months for retinopathy (see pp184–185). All your medication will be reviewed. You may be offered special scans to check your baby's growth and development.

What will happen to my diabetes during labour?

If your labour progresses normally, you may be able to monitor your own blood glucose level and give yourself insulin. If you have been advised not to eat – in case you might need a general anaesthetic – you may need to have an intravenous glucose drip and insulin (see p145) to keep your blood glucose in the recommended range.

Can I breastfeed if I have diabetes?

Yes, although you may be more prone to hypos if you take insulin. Reducing your dose or increasing the amount of carbohydrate food you eat can be helpful. While you are breastfeeding, keep your hypo treatments and snacks nearby and drink extra sugar-free fluid. Taking tablets for diabetes is not recommended while you are breastfeeding.

Caring for someone with diabetes

Q My partner has diabetes. How will this affect our relationship?

Your partner may want you to be closely involved with his or her diabetes care, or may want to manage it alone. Discuss with your partner the type of support he or she needs and wants. On a practical level, it is useful to know what to do if your partner has a hypo (if they take insulin-stimulating tablets or insulin) or what to do if he or she becomes very ill.

Q My parents live in sheltered housing. Although they are well, I worry about them having hypos. How can I make sure they are safe?

Checking what your parents know about hypos and how to treat themselves and each other will help to reassure you about their understanding. If they are unsure of what to do in the event of a hypo, getting information for them might help. Your parents may find that eating regularly is sufficient to prevent hypos most of the time. Having hypo remedies close to hand and checking their blood glucose levels regularly will mean that they are prepared if a hypo happens. If your parents start to have regular hypos, they may need a change of medication.

Q I care full-time for my husband who has diabetes and heart disease. Can I get any help?

Caring for someone full-time can be physically and emotionally demanding – help might be available from friends, family, health professionals, voluntary organizations, and social workers. There might also be a carers' support group in your area which you may find helpful to contact.

Q Our 18-year-old son has diabetes and learning difficulties. How can we help him look after his diabetes?

You may find your son is keener to do some things than others, and he may behave responsibly on one day but not on the next. Forcing him to look after his diabetes when he isn't ready might cause a lot of unnecessary stress for all the family. On the other hand, doing everything for him might feel like a lot of hard work. You might strike a balance by encouraging your son to do the things that he is willing and able to do (and always giving him plenty of praise when he does something well) and taking over his diabetes care when he is struggling.

Q My husband and son both have diabetes. My son is also obese. I'm fed up with making three different meals a day. What can I do?

The guidelines for eating healthily are the same for all three of you, but you may have different tastes in food. Rather than diabetes being the reason to prepare different foods, it might help you to discuss as a family the foods each of you like and how to include these. If your son needs to lose weight, but your husband does not, you may be able to adjust the portion sizes of meals so that your son eats fewer calories than your husband (see pp72–73 for more information on calories).

Q My teenage daughter has just been diagnosed with diabetes, but won't seem to accept it. What can I do?

Your daughter might have strong feelings about her diagnosis; these may range from denial to anger, resentment, and depression. She may also be feeling very self-conscious about her body if she is overweight. You might help your daughter by giving as much emotional support as you can, while also being firm and consistent in your approach to her diabetes care. If you are finding it difficult to communicate with her, your daughter might talk more easily with another member of the family, a friend, or a counsellor.

Living with someone with diabetes

Q My child has been diagnosed with Type 2 diabetes. How will I cope?

You may have experienced a variety of emotions when you discovered that your child had diabetes. You may feel angry, upset, guilty, helpless, or anxious. Your health professional can provide you with information about any local support networks and put you in touch with others in a similar position. Learning more about diabetes can also reassure you that you have the most up-to-date information to help you care for your child.

Q How do I look after my child with Type 2 diabetes?

Helping your child to choose healthy food options, and encouraging them to do lots of physical activity and lose weight will help to keep them healthy. Blood glucose testing, taking prescribed medication, and attending diabetes clinics are all part of routine diabetes care for children as well as adults. Your health professional can advise you about specific aspects of diabetes care, for example, coping with diabetes at school or when your child is away from home.

Q I live with my 85-year-old mother who has just been diagnosed with diabetes. How will I need to help her?

Your mother may have symptoms such as blurred vision, intense thirst, or passing urine frequently, and she may need you to read things for her, and help her to get drinks, or visit the toilet. When her blood glucose is lower, her symptoms will abate but she may need to test her blood glucose and take medication. You can also help her to eat healthy food on a regular basis.

I don't feel that my husband looks after his diabetes properly. Is it right to interfere?

Discovering what your husband thinks about how well he is looking after his diabetes – and listening to him impartially – is more helpful than directly interfering. Being interested and learning more about diabetes will help you to be aware of the issues your husband might be facing. Helping him to find his own solutions is more likely to be successful in the long term than offering advice. In particular, being critical can lead to mutual resentment and make it less easy for the two of you to have an objective discussion about his diabetes.

I'm frightened I won't be able to cope if my girlfriend develops complications. What can I do?

Finding out with your girlfriend about the long-term complications of diabetes, what causes them, and how to help prevent them, will increase your confidence. There is a lot that your girlfriend might be able to do on a day-to-day basis to look after her health. If she is happy for you to attend her annual review (see pp120–121), you can go along and ask her health professional about any issues that are worrying you. If your girlfriend does develop long-term complications, understanding what treatment she needs – and how she should care for her diabetes – means you can give support and assistance where necessary.

I'm always worried about whether my partner has done his tests and injections. How can I cope better?

Worrying about someone close to you is normal. Sharing your concerns with your partner and avoiding blaming him or being critical will help you both to find solutions. Find out whether he would like to be reminded about blood glucose tests and injections, or whether he would feel that you were checking up on him. See pp38–41 for more information on dealing with the emotional aspects of diabetes.

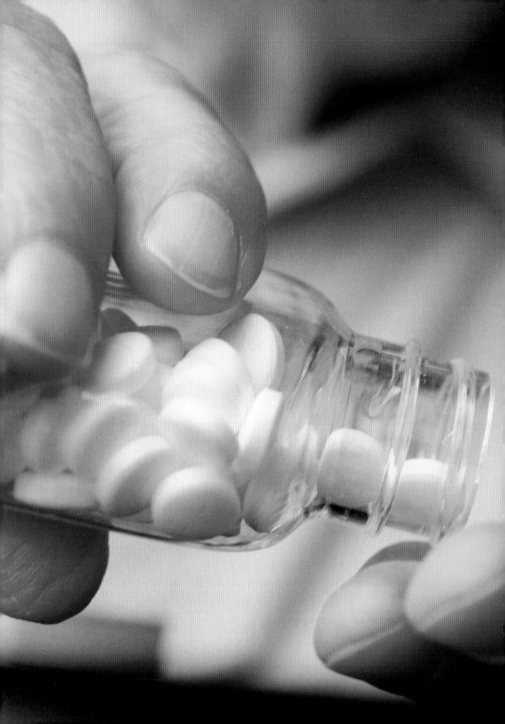

Medication

You will probably need to take some form of medication to help control your blood glucose level. This medication may take the form of glucose-lowering tablets or insulin injections. You are also likely to need to take tablets for high blood pressure and high blood fat levels, to reduce your risk of circulatory conditions such as heart attack and stroke.

Taking tablets

Q After 3 years of having diabetes I now need tablets to control my glucose level. Is this because I haven't lost enough weight?

When you have Type 2 diabetes, your body cells are resistant to the action of insulin, so your pancreas needs to work harder to produce extra insulin. Eventually, you may no longer produce enough insulin, and then you need tablets to control your blood glucose level. Losing weight reduces your insulin resistance so you can delay your need for tablets, but it is unlikely to stop you needing them entirely.

Q Are the tablets I take for my glucose levels the same as insulin?

No, insulin would be destroyed during digestion before it could reach your bloodstream if taken in tablet form. This is why, if you need insulin, it is taken in the form of injections.

Q Can tablets cure my diabetes?

No, tablets don't cure diabetes. Instead, they work in various ways to help keep your blood glucose in the recommended range. This may seem like a cure but if you stop taking your tablets, your blood glucose will start to rise again.

Q Every 6 months, my health professional seems to prescribe more glucose-lowering tablets. Why is this?

Your diabetes is a progressive condition, which means that it will continually change because your insulin production steadily reduces. The dose and type of tablets may need to be altered to reflect what is happening in your body. Your health professional will prescribe the number and dose of tablets – or insulin – that you need to keep your blood glucose level in the recommended range, and this is likely to continue to change over time.

What is the maximum number of tablets I will need?

Having Type 2 diabetes means that you are likely to have a combination of insulin resistance (causing your blood glucose level to rise), high blood pressure, high blood fat levels, and an increased risk of heart disease. You are likely to need different tablets at different times to treat each aspect of your diabetes, so there is no maximum amount.

Can I adjust the dose of my glucose-lowering tablets myself?

Knowing how your tablets work, for how long, and what the maximum dose is makes it more likely that you can make your own dose adjustments successfully. You may find this useful when you are ill or if your routine changes frequently. Regular blood glucose testing will tell you whether your adjustments have achieved the result you wanted. Keep your health professional informed about changes you've made.

What should I do if I forget to take a tablet?

If you remember within the hour, take the tablet then. If you forget until the next tablet is due, take your usual dose rather than taking double. If you forget a tablet occasionally, this is unlikely to do you any harm, but if you are constantly forgetting, you may need to find ways of reminding yourself (see below).

I need three different types of tablet – how can I remember to take them all?

Count out your tablets at the beginning of the day and check you have taken them all at the end of the day. You can also put your tablets somewhere obvious, for example, by the kettle or on a bedside table. You could set an alarm for the time you need to take your tablets or ask someone to remind or call you. If you are often away from home at the times when you take your tablets, keep a supply in your pocket or bag.

TABLETS TO TREAT RAISED BLOOD GLUCOSE

You may be prescribed one or more of these drugs to control your blood glucose level. Some tablets contain a combination of two of the drugs shown – this helps to reduce the number of tablets you need to take. Your health professional will know which tablets are available in combination form.

TYPE OF DRUG	BIGUANIDE
Example	Metformin
How it works	Increases body cells' sensitivity to insulin, and reduces amount of glucose produced by your liver.
Dosage and timing	500mg and 850mg tablets. The initial dose is a single tablet (500mg); the maximum dose is 1g three times a day. You need to take it with or after meals. Slow-release tablets (once a day) are also available.
Precautions/other information	Side effects include nausea and diarrhoea, which can be reduced by taking your tablets with or after a meal, starting with a small dose and increasing gradually, or taking slow-release tablets. If you have kidney problems or severe heart disease, metformin may not be suitable for you.

TYPE OF DRUG	SULPHONYLUREAS
Examples	Gliclazide, glibenclamide, and glimepiride
How they work	Increase your insulin production.
Dosage and timing	Once, twice, or three times a day before meals, depending on your tablets' duration of action.
Precautions/other information	Side effects include weight gain and hypos. You may need to eat regular meals or snacks to avoid hypos. If you also take other drugs, for example non-steroidal anti-inflammatory drugs (NSAIDs) – or if you are pregnant or breastfeeding, or have reduced kidney or liver function, you may not be able to take sulphonylureas.

TYPE OF DRUG	THIAZOLIDINEDIONES (GLITAZONES)
Examples	Rosiglitazone and pioglitazone
How they work	Reduce your insulin resistance and have a beneficial effect on blood fat levels, helping to protect against heart disease.
Dosage and timing	Once a day; either one or two tablets at a time.
Precautions/other information	Side effects include putting on weight and retaining fluid. If you have heart failure or reduced liver function, you are pregnant or breastfeeding, or you are taking tablets to remove extra fluid in your body, these tablets will not be suitable for you. You may need regular liver function tests.

TYPE OF DRUG	MEALTIME GLUCOSE REGULATORS
Examples	Repaglinide and nateglinide
How they work	Increase your insulin production over a short period.
Dosage and timing	One tablet before each meal.
Precautions/other information	Gaining weight and hypos are possible side effects but less likely than with other insulin-stimulating tablets because they work just at mealtimes. If you are pregnant or breastfeeding they are unsuitable for you.

TYPE OF DRUG	ALPHA-GLUCOSIDASE INHIBITOR
Example	Acarbose
How it works	Slows down speed at which carbohydrate is digested and absorbed so that glucose is released more slowly into your bloodstream.
Dosage and timing	25–50mg once a day with the first mouthful of your evening meal, increased slowly every 2–3 weeks up to a maximum of 200mg three times a day with meals.
Precautions/other information	Side effects include flatulence and diarrhoea. If you are pregnant or breastfeeding, it is unsuitable for you.

TABLETS FOR HIGH BLOOD PRESSURE

You will probably need more than one type of tablet to control your blood pressure. Taking small doses of tablets in combination rather than large doses of single tablets can limit side effects. When you first take tablets, you are likely to take a small dose at night (to prevent your blood pressure dropping when you stand up). Your dose will be increased until it controls your blood pressure effectively.

TYPE OF DRUG	ACE (ANGIOTENSIN CONVERTING ENZYME) INHIBITORS
Examples	Lisinopril, captopril, enalapril, perindopril, and ramipril
How they work	These drugs relax blood vessels to lower your blood pressure. They also lower pressure on the filtering units in your kidneys; they help prevent further kidney damage if you have early nephropathy.
Precautions/other information	The main side effect is a dry cough. They may be less effective if you are of African–Caribbean origin. They may not be suitable if you have autonomic neuropathy, are pregnant, or take diuretic tablets, such as amiloride or spironolactone.

TYPE OF DRUG	ANGIOTENSIN II RECEPTOR ANTAGONISTS
Examples	Losartan, irbesartan, valsartan, and candesartan
How they work	They relax your blood vessels, lowering your blood pressure and lower the pressure of blood flowing through your kidneys.
Precautions/other information	You may be prescribed these instead of ACE inhibitors if you have a cough as a side effect (see above).

TYPE OF DRUG	ALPHA 1 BLOCKERS
Examples	Doxazosin, prazosin, and hydralazine
How they work	Widen blood vessels to help your blood flow more easily. They can also reduce blood fat levels and insulin sensitivity.
Precautions/other information	You may experience a blocked nose or low blood pressure on standing as side effects.

TYPE OF DRUG	BETA BLOCKERS
Examples	Atenolol, metoprolol, and propranolol
How they work	They block the action of adrenaline (a hormone that causes your blood vessels to narrow). Some beta blockers act directly on your heart, reducing the amount of blood it pumps at a time.
Precautions/other information	Beta blockers are not suitable if you have asthma or peripheral ischaemia (see p191). Side effects you may experience include less warning of hypos, cold hands, vivid dreams, and a rise in blood glucose and blood fats. If you are male you may develop erectile dysfunction. Beta blockers may be less effective if you are of African–Caribbean origin.

TYPE OF DRUG	CALCIUM CHANNEL BLOCKERS
Examples	Nifedipine, amlodipine, diltiazem, and verapamil
How they work	They lower your blood pressure by dilating (widening) your blood vessels.
Precautions/other information	These might be prescribed if you have angina or an irregular heartbeat (arrhythmia) as well as high blood pressure. Side effects include fluid retention in your ankles. Calcium channel blockers are not suitable if you have heart failure or autonomic neuropathy (see p199).

TYPE OF DRUG	DIURETICS
Examples	Furosemide, bendroflumethiazide, and indapamide
How they work	They increase the amount of fluid your kidneys excrete (so lowering blood pressure by reducing the amount of fluid throughout your body) and dilate (widen) your blood vessels.
Precautions/other information	These drugs may help protect you from a stroke. They may cause your blood glucose level and blood fat levels to rise and can contribute to erectile dysfunction (see pp196–197).

OTHER TABLETS YOU MAY BE PRESCRIBED

In addition to tablets for your blood glucose and your blood pressure, you may also be prescribed tablets if you have other conditions related to your Type 2 diabetes. This chart gives you information about some of the tablets that you may be prescribed for these conditions.

TYPE OF TABLET	ASPIRIN
How it works	Aspirin makes your blood clot less readily, making it flow through your blood vessels more efficiently.
Dosage and timing	You are likely to be prescribed a small dose of aspirin (up to 300mg) each day using the coated variety and be recommended to take it with food.
Precautions/other information	If you do not already take aspirin regularly, you may be given it if you are suspected of having a heart attack. Aspirin may also be recommended if you are flying long distances, unless you are known to have side effects from it. You would not be prescribed aspirin if you have a stomach ulcer or abnormal bleeding patterns as it can irritate your stomach lining. An alternative may be prescribed if aspirin is unsuitable for you.

TYPE OF TABLET	STATINS
Examples	Atorvastatin, pravastatin, and simvastatin
How they work	Statins work by reducing the level of total cholesterol and LDL cholesterol in your bloodstream. Some also reduce the level of triglycerides in your blood.
Dosage and timing	You are likely to be prescribed a single dose of statin to take once a day at any time.
Precautions/other information	You will need to have your liver function checked before starting treatment with a statin and regularly while you are taking it. You may experience stomach ache, indigestion, constipation, and flatulence as side effects.

TYPE OF TABLET	FIBRATES
Examples	Bezafibrate, gemfibrozil, and fenofibrate
How they work	Fibrates work by reducing the amount of triglycerides in your bloodstream and by increasing your HDL cholesterol.
Dosage and timing	You will be prescribed a single dose of fibrate each day.
Precautions/other information	You will have your kidney function checked before starting a fibrate. Some statins cannot be used in combination with fibrates.

TYPE OF TABLET	PANCREATIC LIPASE INHIBITOR
Example	Orlistat
How it works	It reduces your body's ability to process fat, so that it passes through your body.
Dosage and timing	You take one tablet with each meal, up to three a day.
Precautions/other information	You may be prescribed this tablet if you are very overweight but you have started to lose weight. It is most successful if you also eat healthily and try to reduce the amount of calories you are eating. You may experience side effects including flatulence and a sense of urgency in your bowel movements and diarrhoea. If you continue to lose weight using orlistat, you may find your blood glucose and cholesterol levels also reduce.

TYPE OF TABLET	APPETITE SUPPRESSANTS
Example	Sibutramine
How they work	These tablets work by reducing your appetite and slightly increasing your body temperature so you burn more calories.
Dosage and timing	You take one tablet each day.
Precautions/other information	Sibutramine can be successful in helping you to lose weight but your blood pressure may rise so you will have regular blood pressure checks while you are taking it.

The role of insulin injections

Q I've taken tablets for my diabetes for years. Why do I need to start injecting insulin?

Your natural insulin production is so low that, even with the help of tablets, eating healthily, and being active, your blood glucose is not adequately controlled. Your blood glucose tests and HbA1c test will show that your blood glucose level is persistently higher than the recommended range of 4–7 millimoles per litre.

Q I usually take tablets. Why was I given insulin when I went into hospital?

When you are unwell or stressed, your blood glucose level can rise. Keeping your glucose level within the recommended range is an important part of your recovery, so if you need a major operation or are too ill to eat or drink, you will need insulin temporarily by infusion (see p145) or by injection. If you have had a heart attack, you may be prescribed insulin by injection for some months, even after you leave hospital.

Q Does the insulin I inject work in the same way as insulin produced naturally?

Yes, it lowers the level of glucose in your blood by enabling your body cells to take in glucose, and your liver and muscles to store glucose in the form of glycogen. Insulin also plays an important part in preventing glycogen in your liver from being converted back into glucose.

Q Can I stop taking tablets now I'm on insulin?

Not necessarily – your health professional might suggest that you continue taking some or all of your tablets as well as insulin. This is because your tablets can help your body to use the insulin you inject as effectively as possible. See pp158–159 for information on how your glucose-lowering tablets work.

What is the maximum dose of insulin?

Unlike other medications, such as painkillers or antibiotics, there is no maximum dose of insulin. Everyone's needs are different and your insulin dose will vary according to your blood glucose level. You may start by taking a small dose (10–20 units per day) of insulin, but this may gradually increase and vary until you find the dose that keeps your blood glucose in the recommended range of 4–7 millimoles per litre.

Does insulin have any side effects?

Insulin will cause a hypo if it is not balanced with carbohydrate-containing food or if your dose is higher than you need. Also, one of insulin's functions is to enable your body to store glucose, so it can cause weight gain. Rarely, the preservatives in insulin can cause an allergic reaction. In this case, you can try an insulin with different additives. Your health professional will be able to prescribe a type of insulin that suits you.

NORMAL BLOOD GLUCOSE AND INSULIN LEVELS

Your pancreas maintains a background level of insulin and produces extra insulin to deal with rises in blood glucose when you eat and drink.

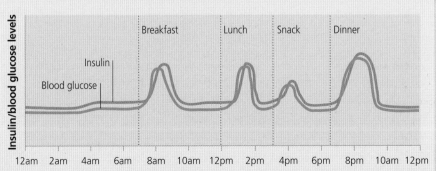

TYPES OF INSULIN

There are several types of insulin, grouped according to how quickly they act and how long they work. Rapid- and short-acting insulins have a quick onset and a short duration of action. They are used at mealtimes to deal with the rise in your blood glucose that eating brings. You can have extra doses if necessary. Intermediate-acting, long-acting, and peakless long-acting insulins are released into your bloodstream slowly and provide a constant background level of insulin.

TYPE OF INSULIN	RAPID-ACTING INSULIN
Brand names	NovoRapid, Humalog, and Apidra
When taken	Just before meals or up to 15 minutes afterwards.
Peak of action	Between 1 and 2 hours.
Duration of action	Up to 5 hours.
Comments	Less chance of hypos than with short-acting insulin because it wears off more quickly. Insulin pumps usually use rapid-acting insulin.

TYPE OF INSULIN	SHORT-ACTING INSULIN
Brand names	Humulin S, Insuman Rapid, and Hypurin Neutral
When taken	20–30 minutes before meals.
Peak of action	Between 2 and 3 hours.
Duration of action	Up to 8 hours.
Comments	You may need a snack 2–3 hours after a meal to avoid a hypo.

TYPE OF INSULIN	INTERMEDIATE-ACTING INSULIN
Brand names	Humulin I, Insulatard, Insuman Basal, and Hypurin Isophane
When taken	Morning, evening, or both (no need to take with food).
Peak of action	Between 4 and 8 hours.
Duration of action	Up to 20 hours.
Comments	You may need a snack around the peak of action, late morning, and before bed, to prevent hypoglycaemia.

TYPE OF INSULIN	LONG-ACTING INSULIN
Brand names	Hypurin Protamine Zinc
When taken	Once a day, usually evening.
Peak of action	Between 6 and 10 hours.
Duration of action	Up to 24 hours.
Comments	The long duration of action can increase your risk of hypoglycaemia.

TYPE OF INSULIN	PEAKLESS LONG-ACTING INSULIN
Brand names	Lantus and Detemir
When taken	At 24-hour intervals.
Peak of action	None.
Duration of action	Approximately 24 hours.
Comments	Reduces your chance of hypos because there is no peak of action.

TYPE OF INSULIN	MIXED INSULINS
Brand names	• Those containing short-acting insulin: Mixtard 10 (or 20, 30, 40, 50), Humulin M2 (or M3, M5), Insuman Comb 15 (or 25, 50), Hypurin Porcine 30/70 mix • Those containing rapid-acting insulin: Humalog Mix25 (or Mix50), NovoRapid 30
When taken	Twice a day, with your breakfast and evening meal. If your brand contains short-acting insulin, 20–30 minutes before your meal. If it contains rapid-acting insulin, just before or up to 15 minutes after your meal.
Comments	These insulins are a mixture of two types of insulin, either rapid- or short-acting insulin plus intermediate- or long-acting insulin. The peak and duration of action are a combination of both insulins. Because of this, you might need snacks between meals and before bed.

Insulin regimens

Q What is an insulin regimen?

This is the term used to describe the type(s) of insulin you inject and how many injections you need a day. Your insulin regimen ensures you have enough insulin to keep your blood glucose in the recommended range of 4–7 millimoles per litre, including at mealtimes.

Q Will I always have the same insulin regimen?

Not necessarily – you may need to change to a different regimen if you find that you can't keep your blood glucose level within the recommended range, or if you need more flexibility in your daily routine. Lifestyle changes, such as a new job or a major illness, can also alter the type, timing, and amount of insulin you need.

Q Can I start with just one injection a day?

Possibly. Starting with a single bedtime injection prevents your blood glucose rising too much overnight, and taking it once a day also gives you a chance to get used to injections.

Q If I've had diabetes for a long time, will I need more injections every day?

The number of injections you have depends on how well your insulin regimen suits your lifestyle and keeps your blood glucose level in the recommended range. One injection may be enough to do this or you may need up to four injections a day.

Q I've heard there are insulin pumps available – what are they?

Instead of daily injections you may be able to take insulin by means of a pump. This constantly delivers rapid-acting insulin via a tube in your abdomen. You then programme the pump to deliver extra doses at mealtimes and when your blood glucose rises too high.

TYPES OF INSULIN REGIMEN

How often you take your insulin depends on the type of insulin you have been prescribed. You and your health professional will discuss the most appropriate regimen for you.

	ONCE A DAY
Type of insulin	Intermediate-, long-, or peakless long-acting.
Time of injection	Usually before bed but you can take it in the morning.
Comments	This is usually a starting regimen, particularly if you are still producing some insulin yourself.

	TWICE A DAY
Type of insulin	Intermediate-acting, or a mixture of intermediate- plus rapid- or short-acting insulin.
Time of injection	With breakfast and evening meal – exact timing depends on whether you take rapid- or short-acting insulin (see p166).
Comments	Easier to manage if you have a regular lifestyle. If you take an insulin mixture, you will probably need extra snacks mid-morning and before bed to avoid hypos.

	FOUR TIMES A DAY
Type of insulin	One intermediate-, long-, or peakless long-acting insulin injection, plus rapid- or short-acting injections before meals.
Time of injection	Longer-acting – usually before bed, but can be in the morning. Shorter-acting – with meals (exact timing depends on whether you take rapid- or short-acting insulin; see p166).
Comments	This is the most flexible regimen (apart from using an insulin pump) as you can alter the timing and/or amount of insulin you inject to suit variations in your day. Unlike a mixed insulin regimen, you can alter the doses of your longer- or shorter-acting insulins independently of each other.

Adjusting your insulin doses

Q How will I know if my insulin dose needs adjusting?

Your home blood glucose test results will reveal when your blood glucose is outside the recommended range of 4–7 millimoles per litre, or your target range. If your blood glucose is too high or too low, identifying the cause – for example, being less active, missing a meal, or altering your routine – will help you decide whether to change your food, physical activity, or your insulin dose.

Q Should I consult my health professional if I want to adjust my insulin dose?

When you first start insulin treatment, you will probably need to learn from your health professional about how to alter doses based on your blood glucose test results. Over time, you're likely to gain confidence and be able to make your own adjustments.

Q How do I decide which insulin dose to adjust?

The first step is to identify the time (or times) of day when your blood glucose is too high or low. Then, work out which insulin has its peak effect at that time. For example, if you inject insulin four times a day and your blood glucose is high late in the morning, your breakfast insulin dose needs adjusting. You may need to experiment – you can change it back if it doesn't work.

Q How do I decide how many units to add or take away from my insulin dose?

Making small, gradual changes every day or two, for example, 2–4 units at a time, will increase your chances of achieving your aim without the risk of getting very high or low blood glucose readings. However, if you usually take large doses of insulin, such as 40–60 units in a single dose, you may need to make larger changes, perhaps 4–6 units at a time, to see the effect.

How should I adjust my insulin dose if I am eating out?

If you are eating later than usual, try delaying the timing of your insulin injection to coincide with your meal, and, if you are eating more food than usual, you can also increase your dose. Your blood glucose test results will tell you if your adjustments have worked.

How should I adjust my insulin dose if I'm being more active than usual?

Your blood glucose level falls when you are more active, so you may need to decrease your insulin dose to avoid a hypo. If your activity is unplanned, you can have an extra snack before the activity. Testing your blood glucose later will show whether your action has worked.

How should I adjust my insulin dose when I am ill?

Your blood glucose level is likely to rise when you are ill (see pp142–145). Increasing your insulin dose to keep your glucose level below 10 millimoles per litre will help. This increase may be 2–4 units or more. If you are very ill, you may need several dose increases before your test results are below 10 millimoles per litre. Consult your health professional promptly if your blood glucose level keeps rising despite your actions.

I need to fast at Ramadan. How should I alter my insulin dose?

You are likely to need a reduced dose during fasting. If you still produce your own insulin, you may be able to stop insulin altogether during the fasting hours. Work out with your health professional in advance how to manage your insulin.

How do I know if I've altered my insulin dose enough?

Testing your blood glucose level after any adjustments will inform you about the effect of your dose changes. Unless you're injecting insulin four times a day or using an insulin pump, you will need to wait 2–3 days between adjustments to see if your change has worked.

Insulin equipment

Q **There's such a wide range of injection devices. How do I choose?**

You may find it more convenient to use a disposable device, or prefer a reusable one. Other features that might influence you are how easy you find the device to use, or which type of insulin you are having – not all types of insulin fit in all devices.

Q **How do injection devices work?**

They hold 300 units of insulin and consist of a plunger and a dose-dialling system and a disposable needle. Your device may be disposable, or reusable (you fit an insulin cartridge into reusable devices).

Q **How big are the needles on injection devices?**

You attach the needles yourself and they are small and fine, and range from 5–12.7mm in length. The length you use depends upon what you find most comfortable, and how much fat you have under your skin – the less fat, the shorter the needle.

Q **How does the needle-free device work?**

A needle-free jet injector sends a fine stream of insulin through your skin under pressure. If you are nervous about needles, this device might be useful. You draw up insulin from a bottle each time you need a dose.

Q **What is an insulin pump?**

This is a small electronic device that you can wear all the time. It uses rapid- or short-acting insulin. To use a pump, you need to insert a needle or small plastic tube into your abdomen and attach it to the pump. This gives you small doses of insulin continuously. You can press buttons to deliver extra doses when you eat or when your blood glucose level is too high.

Do I always need to keep insulin in the fridge?

Your current insulin can safely be kept at room temperature (up to 25°C) for a maximum of one month. Your spare insulin supplies should be kept in a fridge at a temperature of 2–8°C. Insulin that is frozen, exposed to high temperatures or direct sunlight, or is out-of-date works less effectively and should be thrown away.

Can I use the same needle for more than one injection?

Syringes with integral needles, and attachable needles for insulin devices, are designed to be used once only. Reused needles can bend or become blunt and, with reused syringes, the markings may wear off over time.

How can I safely dispose of my needles?

You can use a small, portable needle-clipping device to clip the ends off your used needles. Alternatively, you can use a sharps box to store them. Both of these are available on prescription.

TYPES OF INSULIN EQUIPMENT

There are several different types of device you can use to deliver insulin. A standard insulin device is often pen-shaped and can be reused, or you may prefer to inject using a disposable syringe. No single device is more accurate than another. Your health professional will work with you to find the device that best suits you and your lifestyle.

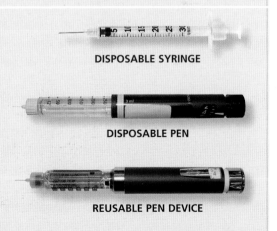

DISPOSABLE SYRINGE

DISPOSABLE PEN

REUSABLE PEN DEVICE

Injecting yourself

Q What checks should I carry out before I inject myself?

Before you inject insulin, check its appearance and expiry date. If it is cloudy when it should be clear, or if it has a pink tinge, looks lumpy, or contains particles after you have rotated it, discard it and use new insulin.

Q I've been told I need to take insulin – do I have to inject into a vein?

No, you insert the needle into the fat beneath your skin (the subcutaneous layer) and the insulin is absorbed from here into your bloodstream. You may occasionally bleed when you inject, but using the recommended sites (see opposite), will help you avoid this.

Q I've got lumpy areas in my abdomen. It's less painful to inject there but I've been told not to – why?

If you repeatedly inject into one site, the constant presence of insulin builds up the fat cells and causes lumps to form (see lipohypertrophy; p198). Injecting into a lumpy site means that insulin will enter your bloodstream less efficiently and make your blood glucose level erratic.

Q How do I give myself an injection?

Follow the steps in the box on p176 or p177. If you are using 12.7mm needles, or if you are using 8mm needles but have very little fat under your skin, you will need to pinch up your skin between your thumb and index finger. Then insert your needle at an angle of 90 degrees and inject. After 10 seconds, remove the needle and release your skin. This technique prevents you from accidentally injecting into muscle. If you use 5mm or 6mm needles, or if you use 8mm needles and you have a deep layer of fat under your skin, you can insert the needle at 90 degrees without pinching up your skin.

Q How can I make injections as comfortable as possible?

Being relaxed and trying not to tense your muscles when you are about to inject can make it more comfortable. Using the pinch-up technique, if this is appropriate for you, will also help (see p176). Insulin that is at room temperature is less likely to cause you discomfort than insulin that you have taken straight from the refrigerator. Using a new needle every time you inject also makes your injection more comfortable. If your injections are always uncomfortable despite these tips, try a shorter needle prescribed by your health professional.

INSULIN INJECTING SITES

Knowing where to inject your insulin is important. The coloured areas on these diagrams are the areas on your body into which you can safely inject. The upper outer arms can be used, with guidance from your health professional about the correct size needle to use. In other areas, there is less subcutaneous fat, so you would be more likely to inject into muscle. You need to change your injection sites every few days to avoid lumps forming. Even if you inject into one site more than others, injecting over a wide area within that site will reduce this risk.

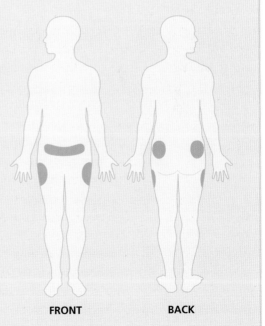

FRONT　　　　**BACK**

HOW TO USE AN INSULIN DEVICE

Whether your insulin device is reusable or disposable, it works in the same way, although the details may vary slightly from one device to another – reading the manufacturer's instructions will tell you exactly how to use it. Check the appearance and expiry date of your insulin before you inject yourself (see p174). This person is using the pinch-up technique.

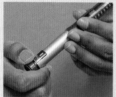

① Pull off the outer cover of your insulin device and screw a needle into the cartridge in its holder. Remove the needle's inner cap. If you are injecting a cloudy insulin, rotate your device (resuspending) to ensure it is uniformly cloudy.

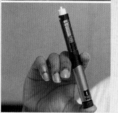

② Dial a small dose of 2–4 units and press the plunger until a drop of insulin appears at the end of the needle. This is called an air shot and it ensures that the plunger is connecting properly and it expels any air from the device. Repeat this step if no insulin appears the first time.

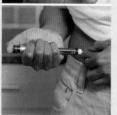

③ Dial the dose that you wish to inject. Then, pinch up a fold of skin at your chosen injection site (in this case, the abdomen). Insert the needle all the way in to your pinched-up skin, making sure the insulin device is at a 90 degree angle to your body.

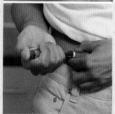

④ Press the plunger and keep it depressed while you inject your dose of insulin. Then, leave the needle in your skin for about 10 seconds (longer if you are injecting a large dose) before removing it. Dispose of your needle if you need to, and replace the cap of your insulin device.

HOW TO USE A SYRINGE

Check the appearance and expiry date of your insulin before you inject yourself. Discard any insulin that is out-of-date or looks different from usual. Make sure that the top of the insulin bottle is clean and use a new syringe each time you inject. This person is using the pinch-up technique (see box opposite).

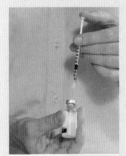

① For cloudy insulin, rotate the bottle (resuspending) so it is uniformly cloudy. Uncap the needle and draw air into the syringe to match the insulin required. Insert the needle into the bottle and inject the air into the bottle. Invert the bottle and check that the needle is in the insulin. Pull back the plunger to draw up insulin. When you have drawn up the correct dose, withdraw the needle from the insulin bottle.

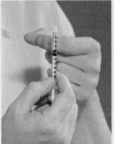

② Remove any air bubbles by holding the syringe with the needle pointing upwards and tapping or flicking the bubbles to the needle end. Gently press on the plunger to push out any air bubbles. Check that you still have the correct dose of insulin in the syringe. Draw up more insulin if you do not have the required dose.

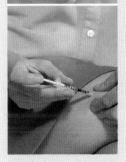

③ Pinch up a fold of skin at your chosen injection site (in this case, the thigh) and insert the needle at a 90 degree angle to your body. Press the plunger to deliver the insulin. After injecting, remove the syringe and dispose of it by putting it into a puncture-proof container known as a sharps box or use a needle-clipping device to clip the needle from the syringe.

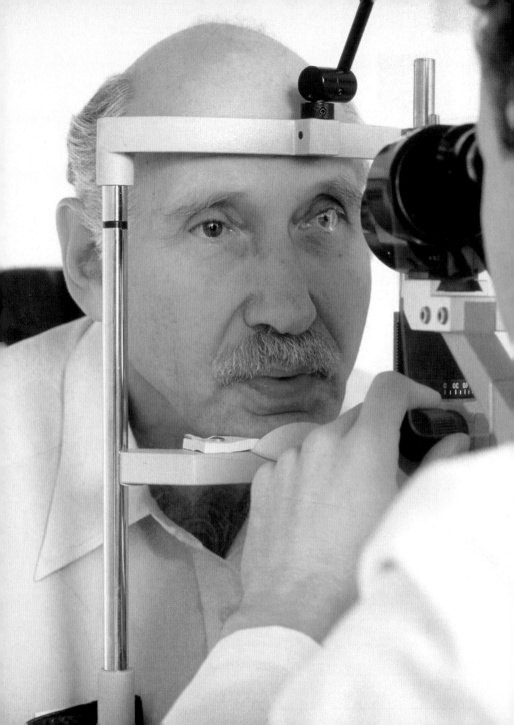

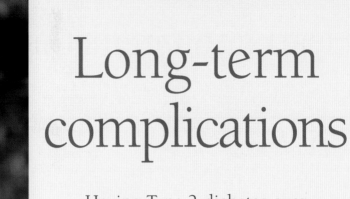

Long-term complications

Having Type 2 diabetes over
a period of years can result in
damage to your blood vessels
and nerves and this can affect
your health in a number of ways,
including your heart and your
circulation. Being aware of these
complications will enable you
to take steps towards preventing
them. Knowing what treatments
are available can be helpful.

Heart and circulatory disease

Q Why am I at risk of heart and circulatory disease?

Type 2 diabetes is strongly linked to high blood pressure and high fat levels in your blood (hyperlipidaemia), which are major risk factors for other conditions, such as coronary heart disease (CHD), stroke, and peripheral vascular disease. Although you will always have diabetes, adopting a healthy lifestyle can reduce your risk of cardiovascular conditions.

Q What can I do to make sure my blood pressure stays under control?

Eating healthily, becoming more active, managing stress, losing weight, and stopping smoking if you need to, can help to lower your blood pressure. Reducing your salt intake (by cutting down on convenience foods and by adding less salt in cooking and at the table) also helps.

Q What treatment will I have for high blood pressure?

As well as the above lifestyle changes, you will probably need tablets. You may be given just one tablet or a combination of three or more (see pp160–161).

Q I've been told I have too much fat in my blood. What does this mean?

You have hyperlipidaemia, which means that your levels of cholesterol or triglycerides are too high (see opposite). This makes you more prone to poor circulation and blocked arteries, which in turn puts you at greater risk of a heart attack or stroke. Drinking less alcohol, choosing monounsaturated rather than saturated fats, and taking more physical activity are all steps you can take to lower your blood fat levels.

What treatment will I have for hyperlipidaemia?

In addition to the actions you can take yourself, you are likely to be prescribed tablets. The particular tablet or tablets that you are given will depend on your blood fat profile. See pp162–163 for information about the types of tablet you might be prescribed.

How would I know if I had coronary heart disease (CHD)?

If you are diagnosed with angina, heart failure, or a heart attack, you have CHD. Angina is a temporary feeling of pain or pressure in your chest, left shoulder, or left arm during stress or exertion. It is caused by your blood circulating less efficiently than usual. Heart failure means that your heart gradually pumps blood around your body less well; signs include swelling in your legs, feet, or around your middle, shortness of breath, and fatigue. Signs of a heart attack include severe chest pain, palpitations, and nausea.

HEALTHY LEVELS OF FATS IN THE BLOOD

High levels of some fats (lipids) in the blood – and low levels of others – increase your risk of coronary heart disease. If you have a blood test to check your lipid levels, these are the results that you need to aim for to keep your heart and blood vessels healthy.

TYPE OF FAT	RECOMMENDED LEVEL
Total cholesterol	Ideally should be below 5.0 millimoles per litre
Triglycerides	Should be less than 2.3 millimoles per litre
LDL cholesterol	Below 2.6 millimoles per litre
HDL cholesterol	Above 1.2 millimoles per litre

Q What treatment will I have for coronary heart disease?

You will be prescribed tablets and you may also need surgery. The type of tablets you might be prescribed are shown in the charts on pp160–163. If you need surgery, you might have a coronary artery bypass or coronary angioplasty. Bypass surgery involves grafting a blood vessel from another part of your body, for example, your leg, and using it to replace the blocked section of the artery supplying your heart. A coronary angioplasty operation widens your partially blocked artery using a tube that is inflated and then removed. You may also have a metal device inserted to permanently hold the artery open.

Q How is a heart attack treated?

If you have a heart attack, you will need to call an ambulance. The ambulance staff will immediately give you aspirin and set up a drip to reduce the risk of your blood clotting. You will be admitted to hospital where you will have an insulin infusion to control your blood glucose level (see p145). You will have treatment for your blood pressure and blood fat levels, and your heart will be monitored closely. Once you have recovered, you will start a cardiac rehabilitation programme. You may be asked to continue insulin injections at home for at least the first few months to reduce your chances of having a further heart attack.

Q Why do I have pain in my calves when I walk?

You may have peripheral vascular disease (PVD). This means the blood vessels supplying your legs become partially blocked. When you walk, your muscles get a limited supply of blood, and this causes you pain. If you have severe PVD, you may only be able to walk very short distances.

Q What treatment will I have for peripheral vascular disease?

You may be prescribed tablets to increase your circulation or the elasticity of your blood vessels (see pp160–161). If your arteries are severely blocked, you may also be offered surgery in the form of angioplasty or a coronary artery bypass (see opposite).

Q What is a stroke?

A stroke, medically known as a cerebrovascular accident (CVA), occurs when the blood flow to your brain is interrupted as a result of a blood clot or a burst blood vessel. Your brain is then deprived of oxygen and some brain cells die or are damaged. A stroke is diagnosed by your symptoms and/or a brain scan. Your recovery depends on the extent to which your brain has been affected. High blood pressure is the main risk factor for a stroke, so keeping your blood pressure in the recommended range (see p117) helps to reduce your risk.

Q What are the symptoms of a stroke?

Depending on which part of your brain is affected, you may experience changes in your movement, speech, memory, vision, hearing, or balance. For example, you may have slurred speech, partial or double vision, dizziness, weakness or paralysis of one arm or leg, or abnormal sensations along one side of your body. Your symptoms appear on the side of your body that is opposite the damaged side of your brain.

Q How is a stroke treated?

Your treatment is based on which specific functions have been affected by the stroke. For example, you may be offered physiotherapy to help you with walking and movement, or speech therapy to help you regain your ability to communicate.

Eye conditions

Q I've been told I have early signs of damage to my eye. How is this linked to my diabetes?

Over a period of years, having raised blood glucose and raised blood pressure can cause the blood vessels in your retina (an area at the back of the eye) to become weak and prone to bleeding. Your body tries to grow new vessels to compensate, but these are also weak and bleed easily. This condition is known as retinopathy.

Q What causes retinopathy?

The blood vessels in your retina are small and thin and easily damaged by constant high blood glucose or blood flowing through them at high pressure. You may have had Type 2 diabetes for some years without knowing it, and during this time some early damage may have already occurred. You can stop retinopathy progressing by lowering your blood glucose and blood pressure.

Q What are the symptoms of retinopathy?

You may not have any symptoms of retinopathy because it develops slowly over years. Your first sign might be a sudden loss of sight due to a bleeding blood vessel in your retina. This is why an annual eye check is vital, as changes can be detected before they affect your sight.

Q Are there stages of retinopathy?

There are three stages: background retinopathy, pre-proliferative retinopathy, and proliferative retinopathy. If you have background retinopathy, your vision does not change, but in the next two stages, when your retina grows new blood vessels and these bleed, you will find your sight is affected to a minor or major degree. If you have pre-proliferative or proliferative retinopathy, you will be offered treatment by laser therapy or surgery.

What would happen if my retinopathy was not treated?

If retinopathy progresses beyond the background stage, eventually your sight may become limited or even lost. This may be caused by one of the complications of retinopathy. These include: maculopathy (affecting your central vision), vitreous haemorrhage (bleeding into the space between your lens and your retina), retinal detachment (causing sudden loss of sight), and rubeotic glaucoma (new blood vessels growing on your iris, the coloured part of your eye).

How is retinopathy diagnosed?

There are a range of tests to check if you have retinopathy. You are asked to read rows of letters on a chart known as a Snellen chart. You also have a digital photograph taken of the backs of your eyes (you may be given eye drops to dilate your pupils before this), and your eyes may be examined using an instrument called an ophthalmoscope. If you have advanced retinopathy, you might have a special examination known as fluorescein angiography, in which a dye is injected into a vein in your arm. The dye travels to the blood vessels in your eye and your retina is then examined under X-ray.

What is the treatment for retinopathy?

This depends on how advanced your condition is. In the early stages (background retinopathy), you don't need any treatment, but your eyes are photographed regularly (every 6 months) for signs of deterioration. If you have a later stage of retinopathy, you will have laser treatment at a specialist outpatient clinic. Laser beams are used to destroy the fragile new blood vessels that have formed. You may also have laser treatment if you have maculopathy or a vitreous haemorrhage.

Myth "My routine sight check will show if diabetes has damaged my eyes"

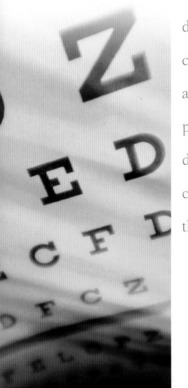

Truth Not necessarily. To check for eye damage due to diabetes, your optician would need to check your eyes in a specific way, by looking at the backs of your eyes or taking a digital photograph of them after your pupils have been dilated (widened) using drops. The routine sight check you have for your glasses will not include these examinations.

Q Can eye surgery restore my vision?

If you have vitreous haemorrhage, rubeotic glaucoma, or retinal detachment, eye surgery can help. In all of these complications, extensive damage has already affected your retina. As with any treatment for advanced retinopathy, your treatment will save as much of your sight as possible.

Q Is it true that I am more prone to cataracts?

Yes, you are more likely to develop cataracts if you have diabetes. A cataract is a clouding over of the lens of your eye.

Q What are the symptoms of cataracts?

You might experience gradual loss of vision because the cloudiness of your lens prevents sufficient light from entering your eye. Also, you might see a "halo" on bright lights.

Q How are cataracts treated?

Cataracts develop slowly and may never require treatment. However, if your vision deteriorates, cataracts can be surgically removed under local anaesthetic, and you will have a new lens inserted. This will restore your vision as long as it is not affected by retinopathy.

Q I can't see as well as before – how can I manage my diabetes tests and injections?

If testing your blood glucose level, taking tablets, injecting yourself with insulin or managing hypos is difficult, ask your health professional about equipment that can make things easier. For example, a blood glucose meter that has a memory will enable someone else to read your test results at a convenient time. An insulin delivery device that provides a fixed dose, or a tablet box with sections for each day, may also help. If your vision is particularly affected, you may need help from someone else to manage your diabetes safely.

Kidney conditions

Q My health professional says I have tiny amounts of protein in my urine. What does this mean?

This may mean that you have the first signs of damage to your kidneys, a condition known medically as nephropathy or renal (kidney) disease. Having high blood pressure and a high blood glucose level over a long period of time (perhaps before your diabetes is diagnosed) can lead to you developing nephropathy. When your nephropathy is detected in this first stage, known as microalbuminuria, lowering your blood pressure and blood glucose level can help to reverse it.

Q How will I know if I have nephropathy?

As part of your diabetes care, your health professional will test your urine once or twice a year to check for the presence of protein (a sign of possible kidney damage). A single positive test for protein does not necessarily mean that you have kidney damage. Urine infections, such as cystitis (see p147), can also cause protein levels in urine to rise. For this reason, if a single test is positive, you will have follow-up tests. If these show that your kidneys are continuously leaking protein, this means you have nephropathy.

Q What are the stages of nephropathy?

There are three main stages: the first stage is microalbuminuria, in which tiny amounts of a protein called albumin are found in your urine; the second is proteinuria, in which a higher quantity of protein is present in your urine and some permanent damage to your kidneys may have occurred. The third stage is end-stage renal failure when your kidneys stop working because they can no longer filter out waste products.

Q What are the symptoms of nephropathy?

You may have no symptoms in the early stages of nephropathy. However, if your body starts to lose protein in large amounts, and you do not receive treatment, your body will retain fluid (making your ankles or legs swell), and you may be short of breath, feel tired, nauseous, and have itchy skin. With end-stage renal failure, your face, limbs, and abdomen may swell, you may lose weight, produce little urine, have very itchy skin, and feel lethargic and nauseous.

Q What is the treatment for nephropathy?

Initially, you will be prescribed ACE inhibitor tablets (see p160), which help to reduce the amount of protein you lose through your kidneys. Your blood pressure will be checked regularly and treated if necessary, and you will have at least twice-yearly blood and urine tests to check your kidney function, as well as twice-yearly HbA1c tests (see pp113–114). You may be asked to drink less fluid and to cut down on protein, potassium, and salt to prevent the build up of waste products. A specialist dietitian will advise you.

Q What is dialysis?

If your kidneys can no longer filter your blood and get rid of waste products, dialysis can carry out this process for you. There are two main forms of dialysis: one is haemodialysis, which involves your blood being pumped through a machine (either in hospital or at home). The other method is peritoneal dialysis, also known as continuous ambulatory peritoneal dialysis (CAPD), which you do yourself every day by running specific fluid through a tube into your abdomen, then draining it off, along with your body's waste products, after several hours.

Foot conditions

Q My health professional says I have peripheral neuropathy. What is this?

It means the nerves supplying the extremities of your body are damaged as a result of a high blood glucose level. Peripheral neuropathy usually causes pain or loss of feeling in your toes and feet, and may affect a small part of one foot, parts of both feet, all of both feet or your lower legs. Rarely, it affects your arms and hands.

Q How would I know if I have peripheral neuropathy?

Symptoms vary according to which type of nerves have been damaged. You may experience: tingling, burning, or prickling; short, stabbing, or burning pains, which are severe at night; numbness or insensitivity to temperature or pain; or extreme sensitivity to touch (even bedclothes). Alternatively, you may have no symptoms, or symptoms may come and go. Your health professional will diagnose neuropathy by assessing your reflexes and your response to light and firm touch.

Q What treatment will I have for peripheral neuropathy?

You may be prescribed tablets. Antidepressants, such as amitriptyline or imipramine, or anticonvulsants, such as gabapentin or carbamazepine, are effective in reducing pain from neuropathy. Creams, such as capsaicin, can also help. If bedclothes irritate your feet and legs, you can apply a film dressing (clingfilm will work) to protect sensitive areas, or you can use a cradle to raise your bedclothes. If your neuropathy progresses, your pain will reduce as your nerves become more damaged. You will need to carefully observe and care for your feet (see p137), and you may need specially-made shoes to protect your feet from excess pressure.

Q Are there any complications of peripheral neuropathy?

Yes, you can develop foot ulcers or a condition known as Charcot foot. If you have neuropathy, your ulcers are most likely to develop on the soles of your feet or on any areas of increased pressure – they can form beneath a layer of hard skin, or be caused by an injury, such as a burn, or a blister from tight or rubbing footwear. Charcot foot is a condition in which the bones in your feet become damaged and distorted.

Q What should I do if I develop a foot ulcer?

You will need urgent treatment, which will include antibiotics. Your health professional will remove any infected tissue, and dress your wound. You will be asked to avoid putting pressure on the ulcer, which may mean wearing a cast on your foot for many weeks. Controlling your blood glucose level will help your ulcer to heal and help prevent it recurring. If it doesn't heal, you may need an amputation of part of your foot.

Q What will happen if I develop Charcot foot?

Your foot will probably become hot, swollen, and painful, getting worse over two to three months. Your bones will be thinner and more easily damaged, for example, fracturing or dislocating your joints, causing your foot shape to alter. Treating Charcot foot involves keeping the weight off affected parts of your feet, usually by wearing a cast in the short-term and specially-made footwear in the long-term.

Q I've been diagnosed with peripheral ischaemia. What is this?

Ischaemia is a condition in which poor circulation, caused by narrowed arteries, means that parts of your body don't get enough oxygen. Your legs and feet are most likely to be affected because they are furthest away from your heart.

Q How can I find out if I have peripheral ischaemia?

Symptoms include: a cramp-like pain in your calves when you walk; cold, pale feet; wounds or injuries that are slow to heal; and persistent foot ulcers. Alternatively, you may not have any symptoms. Your health professional will check your foot pulses as part of your annual review (see pp120–121). Faint or absent pulses are a sign of ischaemia.

Q How is peripheral ischaemia treated?

Your peripheral ischaemia will be regularly monitored by your health professional. If you smoke, it is important to stop (smoking damages your circulation). For severe ischaemia, you may need to have surgery. Your arteries can be widened using a technique called angioplasty, or your damaged blood vessels may need to be bypassed. If surgery is not possible and the blood supply to your foot is blocked, you may need to have an amputation of part or all of your foot or leg.

Q Are there any complications of peripheral ischaemia?

Yes, you may develop foot ulcers and gangrene. The most common site of foot ulcers if you have ischaemia is the side of your foot. It is important to prevent ischaemic ulcers becoming gangrenous – this is when an area of your foot loses its blood supply and the affected tissue dies. Gangrene is treated by amputation of the affected area – this prevents it spreading.

Q Can I develop both peripheral ischaemia and peripheral neuropathy?

Yes, having diabetes makes you prone to both nerve and circulation damage, and your feet and legs are the most likely places to be affected. If you develop both peripheral ischaemia and peripheral neuropathy – known as neuroischaemia – you are also vulnerable to foot ulcers, Charcot foot (see p191), and gangrene.

How can I prevent the complications of ischaemia and neuropathy?

You can check your feet daily for sores or wounds, and take good care of your feet by keeping the area between your toes dry and applying an unperfumed moisturizer to your feet every day. Don't let hard skin build up on your feet and seek prompt help for minor problems such as corns. For more information, see pp135–137.

CHARACTERISTICS OF FOOT CONDITIONS

Peripheral neuropathy and ischaemia cause different problems and have different characteristics. Some people have a combination of these conditions, which further increases your chances of developing foot problems.

PERIPHERAL NEUROPATHY	PERIPHERAL ISCHAEMIA
Warm skin.	Cool or cold skin.
Lack of feeling in foot or feet.	Normal or slightly reduced feeling.
Pink or normal colour.	Pale or blue-tinged colour.
May be painless, but pain can occur and is most severe at night.	Painful during exertion or rest at any time of day.
Normal or increased pulses in the feet.	Faint pulses in the feet, or no pulses at all.
Callused skin.	No callus.
Reduced reflexes.	Normal reflexes.
Prone to ulcers on any areas of pressure, for example, the soles of the feet.	Prone to ulcers on the sides of the feet.
Potential to develop Charcot (misshapen) foot.	Potential to develop gangrene.

Depression

Q What is the link between diabetes and depression?

If you have diabetes, you may be worried about how developing long-term complications will affect your life in the future. Or perhaps you are struggling to manage your day-to-day diabetes routine. Finding it difficult to cope, or not feeling in control of your health, can cause or contribute to depression. In addition, if you are depressed, you might find it hard to stay motivated to look after your diabetes.

Q How can I prevent myself getting depressed?

Anything that makes you feel successful, useful, and in control can help to prevent depression. This may mean spending regular social time with your friends and family, or on your favourite interest or hobby. Work or voluntary work can also give you a sense of self-worth. Being physically active (see pp78–97) helps to prevent or combat depression because it increases the level of mood-enhancing chemicals such as endorphins in your brain. Being aware of the possible signs of depression (see box opposite) and simply talking about how you are feeling from time to time can also help prevent you becoming depressed.

Q How can I help myself feel better when I'm depressed?

Talking to your partner, a friend, or family member can help you to think more clearly about what you are going through. Don't be afraid of asking someone to just listen rather than give you advice. Try to avoid unnecessary pressure when you are feeling low, and be realistic about how much you can achieve. If you have a busy schedule, take time out to do things you enjoy.

Q **How can I manage my diabetes care when I'm feeling depressed?**

Try to set yourself small goals, such as taking your tablets eight or nine times out of 10, or testing your blood glucose just once a day. Asking for help or talking to your health professional is the first step if you find it a challenge to look after yourself.

Q **What treatment can I have for depression?**

Your health professional may recommend counselling, antidepressant tablets, or both. Counselling can help you find new ways of thinking and behaving. Antidepressants work by increasing the levels of one or two chemicals in the brain: serotonin and noradrenaline. Most antidepressants take several weeks to reach their peak effect, which means that you don't feel different immediately. Taking antidepressants for at least six months is recommended.

RECOGNIZING DEPRESSION

These are some of the symptoms of depression. You may have just one symptom or a combination of several.

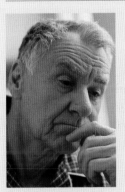

Regularly feeling sad, pessimistic, or hopeless about life, or feeling unable to enjoy things.

Disinterest in your usual activities and relationships.

Feeling anxious or tearful, or crying a lot.

Difficulty sleeping, or waking up very early in the morning.

Feeling constantly lethargic and short of energy.

Finding it difficult to concentrate and feel motivated.

Erection difficulties

Q I've been having trouble getting an erection lately. Could this be linked to my diabetes?

Damage to your blood vessels or nerves as a result of diabetes can affect your ability to get an erection. But erectile dysfunction (ED) can also be a side effect of drugs, such as beta blockers (for high blood pressure). Other causes include: depression, stress, anxiety, relationship difficulties, and heavy smoking and drinking. If your ED is linked to diabetes it will probably develop slowly and you are likely to have difficulty getting an erection at any time of day.

Q How can I find out what's causing my erection difficulties?

You can have a blood pressure check, a physical examination, and a blood test to check your testosterone and thyroxine levels (two hormones that affect sexual response). You may be tested for autonomic neuropathy (see p199) or peripheral neuropathy, conditions that are also caused by nerve damage. You will be asked how much alcohol you drink, and when and how often you get an erection.

Q Is there anything I can do to treat my erection difficulties?

Controlling your blood glucose level as well as you can, stopping smoking if you need to, and reducing your alcohol intake if you drink more than the recommended amount (see pp64–65) can all help.

Q What treatments might I be prescribed?

Apart from tablets (see opposite), there are physical aids that can help you to have an erection, including vacuum devices and penile implants. Asking your health professional about these or contacting a national helpline (see p200) will give you more information.

Q I've become impotent over the last few months – how can I talk to my wife about it?

Enlisting your partner's opinion, help, and support can be valuable, even though ED is a difficult matter to discuss. Explaining to your partner that you find the subject uncomfortable, but that you want her to know what has been happening might make it easier. Discussing how you would both like your sex life to be and talking about the treatments available will help you understand each other's needs.

TABLETS FOR ERECTILE DYSFUNCTION

Several drugs are available to treat erectile dysfunction. These can be prescribed by your doctor – some tablets are not recommended if you take other medication.

DRUG	TIMING/LENGTH OF ACTION	COMMENTS
Sildenafil and vardenafil	One hour before sexual activity. Sildenafil can be effective for up to 6–8 hours; vardenafil for up to 48 hours.	Should not be taken with nitrate drugs (such as isosorbide mononitrate or glyceryl trinitrate), which you might take for angina or high blood pressure – the two drugs combined can cause very low blood pressure.
Tadalafil	Between 30 minutes and 12 hours before sexual activity. It is effective for up to 24 hours.	Should not be taken with nitrate drugs (see above).
Apomorphine hydrochloride	Twenty minutes before sexual activity. It is effective for up to 8 hours.	It is safe to take this drug with nitrates.

Other conditions

Q What other conditions might I develop?

There are two other conditions – lipohypertrophy and autonomic neuropathy – that you could develop if you have diabetes. Lipohypertrophy is a side effect of injecting insulin (you will not develop it if you manage your diabetes with tablets, or with healthy eating and activity). Autonomic neuropathy is a permanent condition that affects the nerves in your body that you cannot consciously control.

Q Why have I got lumps in the place where I inject insulin?

You may have lipohypertrophy. This is the name for fat deposits that accumulate under your skin due to constantly injecting insulin into a small area. You are more likely to get it if you inject into small areas for years, but sometimes it can develop after a few months.

Q What are the symptoms of lipohypertrophy?

If you run your hand over the areas where you inject, you may feel lumps under your skin. You may also find your injections are completely painless – this is because repeated injections in one area damage the nerve supply to your skin. Lipohypertrophy can make your blood glucose levels swing up and down from day to day because your insulin will not be absorbed properly through the lumps under your skin.

Q What can I do about lipohypertrophy?

You can prevent lipohypertrophy by injecting into a slightly different place on each occasion and rotating between the sites on your body you use regularly. If you avoid injecting into lumpy sites, the lumps may lessen or disappear over time.

Q What is autonomic neuropathy?

Autonomic neuropathy is the medical name for damage to nerves that control the parts of your body that you don't move voluntarily. These include the nerves that regulate your temperature, heart rate, and digestion. In men, autonomic neuropathy can affect the nerves that are involved in getting an erection. Autonomic neuropathy can be caused by a blood glucose level that has been consistently high for many years, even before you knew you had diabetes.

Q What are the symptoms of autonomic neuropathy?

You might experience a range of symptoms, depending on which of your nerves are affected. Possible symptoms include: too much or too little sweating; very dry skin; feeling bloated and nauseous, or being sick after you have eaten; diarrhoea or constipation; dizziness when you stand up or get out of bed (this is known as postural hypotension); difficulty being active because your heart rate does not increase or decrease in the normal way; being unable to empty your bladder completely; difficulties in getting an erection; and being less aware of your hypo symptoms.

Q Can I have treatment for autonomic neuropathy?

Your treatment will depend on your symptoms and their severity. Autonomic neuropathy is likely to be permanent, so your treatment will aim to reduce your symptoms. For example, you may be prescribed medication to stop nausea or to control diarrhoea, or you may need an operation to help your stomach empty more efficiently. If you have a tendency to feel faint when you stand up, your health professional will review your blood pressure tablets and consider whether any changes in your treatment would be beneficial.

Useful addresses

British Association for Counselling and Psychotherapy
BACP House, 35–37 Albert Street
Rugby CV21 2SG
Tel: 0870 443 5252
Website: www.bacp.co.uk

Diabetes UK
Macleod House, 10 Parkway,
London NW1 7AA
General enquires: 020 7424 1000
Careline: 0845 120 2960,
or email on careline@diabetes.org.uk
Website: www.diabetes.org.uk

Driver and Vehicle Licensing Agency (DVLA)
DVLA Swansea, SA99 1DL
Tel: 0870 600 0301
Website: www.dvla.gov.uk

National Kidney Federation
6 Stanley Street, Worksop S81 7HX
Tel: 01909 487 795
Website: www.kidney.org.uk

Royal National Institute for the Blind
105 Judd Street, London WC1H 9NE
Tel: 020 7388 1266
Website: www.rnib.org.uk

Sexual Dysfunction Association
Windmill Place Business Centre
2–4 Windmill Lane
Southall UB2 4NJ
Helpline: 0870 7743 571
Website: info@sda.uk.net

Stroke Association
Stroke House,
240 City Road
London EC1V 2PR
Tel: 020 7566 0300
Helpline: 0845 303 3100
Website: www.stroke.org.uk

To contact other people with diabetes, try the following sites:
www.diabetes-insight.info
www.insulin-pumpers.org.uk

For specific information, try:
www.diabetes-exercise.org
www.glycaemicindex.com

Another useful source is the American Diabetes Association
Website: www.diabetes.org

Index

About the Authors

Rosemary Walker and Jill Rodgers worked for many years as diabetes specialist nurses and have been at the forefront of a variety of national initiatives to improve diabetes care. In 2002 they formed their partnership, and now work independently of the NHS as In Balance Healthcare UK. Together, they provide skills-based training for people with diabetes and for health professionals, to make the provision and use of diabetes services more effective and to improve the lives of people with diabetes. Their philosophy is one of empowerment, an approach that acknowledges peoples' ability to make their own decisions about what is right for them. This book and their first book, *Diabetes: A practical guide to managing your health*, have been written using this approach.

Authors' acknowledgments

We would like to thank the people that have helped us shape the content of this book. We particularly wish to acknowledge the many people with diabetes whose thoughts and feelings have given us valuable insight into what helps them live more successfully with their diabetes, Janet Mohun at Dorling Kindersley, our close friends, families and colleagues who have given us much appreciated support and encouragement.

For the publishers

Dorling Kindersley would like to thank Jenny Orr, Amanda Vezey and Emma Bunn at Diabetes UK for their expert advice; Frances Vargo for picture research, Hilary Bird for indexing, and Ann Baggaley for proofreading.

Picture credits

2: Alamy/Stock Connection Distribution/Phoebe Dunn; 7l: Getty Images/FoodPix/Jonelle Weaver, Getty Images/Altrendo Images (c); 8: Corbis/Jose Luis Pelaez, Inc; 22: Corbis/Tom Stewart; 32: Getty Images/Taxi/Adamsmith; 36l: Science Photo Library/Faye Norman; 37: Science Photo Library/BSIP, LENEE; 40: Alamy/Stock Connection Distribution/Lew Lause; 44: Getty Images/PhotoAlto/Jean-Blaise Hall; 50: Anthony Blake Photo Library/J. Lee Studios; 63: Corbis/Michael Keller (t); 76: Corbis/Layne Kennedy; 80: Corbis/Jose Luis Pelaez, Inc; 90: Getty Images/Photonica/White Packert; 91: Getty Images/Taxi/Justin Pumfrey; 97: Getty Images/Photonica/Steve Ibb; 98: Corbis/Steve Prezant; 116: Getty Images/Stone/Charles Thatcher; 122: Corbis/Norbert Schaefer; 134: Getty Images/Taxi/Nick White; 140: Corbis/Chuck Savage; 141: Getty Images/Taxi/Deborah Jaffa; 148: Corbis/Norbert Schaefer; 154: Getty Images/Taxi/Michael Goldman; 178: Science Photo Library/Custom Medical Stock Photo; 186: Getty Images/Stone/Dave Crosier; 195: Corbis/JLP/Sylvia Torres.

All other images © Dorling Kindersley.
For further information see www.dkimages.com